PRAIS

MW00572670

"Allison Alexander's take on being chronically sick is insightful, creative, and engrossing, which makes it hard to put down. She lightens the mood and makes palatable what is normally a very serious subject by weaving together superhero and pop culture references with her unique, humourous voice and keen observations. Unlike most books on the topic, *Super Sick* left me feeling inspired, empowered, and confident that I have much to share with the world, even if I'm not your typical superhero."

— KIRA LYNNE, PROFESSIONAL
COUNSELLOR, PSYCHOTHERAPIST, AUTHOR
OF *ACHES, PAINS, AND LOVE*

"Nothing is off the table in this book and I admired Allison's frankness and honesty about her condition, involving both bladder and bowel, and her journey through dealing with judgement, finding love, managing work, and balancing illness with sexual desires. I highly recommend this refreshing, original and immensely helpful read!"

— JOY H. SELAK, AUTHOR OF *YOU DON'T LOOK SICK! LIVING WELL WITH INVISIBLE CHRONIC ILLNESS*

"Warm and down to earth, *Super Sick* offers real talk about the ordinary heroism of living with a chronic illness—from dating to navigating a medical system that often dismisses women's pain. It is a window into the difficulties of being sick in a culture that valourizes health."

— MAYA DUSENBERY, AUTHOR OF *DOING HARM: THE TRUTH ABOUT HOW BAD MEDICINE AND LAZY SCIENCE LEAVE WOMEN DISMISSED, MISDIAGNOSED, AND SICK*

"Allison writes about the life-altering impact of a serious invisible illness with compelling honesty. A validating read for anyone living with a debilitating illness—and a much-needed course for health care professionals, who still aren't taught how to see the extraordinary expertise our patients bring so that we might support and empower them with dignity and respect."

— VERONIQUE MEAD, MD, MA, BLOGGER AT *CHRONIC ILLNESS TRAUMA STUDIES*

"A must-read for people new to the world of chronic illness."

— JORDAN DAVIDSON, MANAGING EDITOR AT THE MIGHTY

"In her humourous, candid portrayal... [Alexander] provides validation of the soul-sucking, crazy-making medical and life experiences that is the lot of those going through chronic illness. Her memoir runs seamlessly across a gamut of issues from the mundane of daily living to sex and love to the sublime of spiritual and personal development questions, and I cannot imagine going through an experience like hers, or caring for someone that is, and not reading this lovely book."

— KELSEY CROWE, PH. D., CO-AUTHOR OF
*THERE IS NO GOOD CARD FOR THIS: WHAT
TO SAY AND DO WHEN LIFE IS SCARY,
AWFUL, AND UNFAIR TO PEOPLE YOU LOVE*

"More than anything, this book is about courage— the courage to face your fears about your health and the courage to keep fighting for your dignity. Through her personal story (which she shares with refreshing candor and honesty), interviews with others, and examples from cultural superheroes, this special book points the way to making peace with your life no matter what obstacles you face."

— TONI BERNHARD, AUTHOR OF *HOW TO BE
SICK* AND *HOW TO LIVE WELL WITH
CHRONIC PAIN AND ILLNESS*

ISBN 978-1-7770878-2-1 (paperback), 978-1-7770878-3-8 (e-book), 978-1-7770878-4-5 (hardcover), 978-1-7770878-5-2 (large print paperback), 978-1-7770878-6-9 (large print hardcover)

This is a book of nonfiction. The events portrayed are presented to the best of the author's memory and records. Some names and other identifying characteristics of people mentioned in this work have been changed to protect their identities.

Published by Phoenix Quill Press
Winnipeg, Manitoba, Canada
www.aealexander.com

For my mom, who always
came when I called.

SUPER
SICK

Making Peace with Chronic Illness

ALLISON ALEXANDER

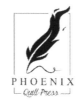

PHOENIX
Quill Press

CONTENTS

FOREWORD

BY FAY ONYX

Being disabled in real life is different from how it's portrayed in fiction. Most fictional representations simultaneously underestimate and overestimate how disability impacts people's lives. These distorted portrayals cast disability as a great tragedy that prevents people from having full, meaningful lives. At the same time, they ignore and minimize the many accessibility barriers that disabled people encounter every day.

Disabled characters overcome barriers with determination and positivity, but in real life, willpower and a positive attitude can't change the harsh reality of accessibility barriers. As Stella Young, a journalist, comedian, and disability activist, said, "No amount of smiling at a flight of stairs has ever made it turn into a ramp. Never. Smiling at a television screen isn't going to make closed captions appear for people who are deaf. No amount of standing in the middle of a bookshop and radiating a positive attitude is going to turn all those books into braille."[1]

Authentic disability representation is needed, as are resources on how to respectfully depict disability. That is how I got started writing about disability—I was struggling to find resources, so I started making them.[2] I began by collecting a list of accessibility resources for gaming, and each time I encountered a gap in the available resources, I did my best to fill it. Over time, this grew into a series of articles on ableist tropes in storytelling, another series on addressing ableism in tabletop role-playing games, a monthly writing advice column for the Mythcreants blog, and a slew of other individual resource pages on my website.

Similarly, I pivoted the focus of my podcast, *Writing Alchemy*, to creating authentic, vivid, and intersectional disability representation. In it, disabled guests and I create stories about disabled heroes using the collaborative storytelling of tabletop role-playing games. This, in turn, led me to create *Magic Goes Awry*, a high fantasy role-playing game that aims to capture the fun of Dungeons and Dragons in a rules-light system that is accessible to a wider range of people.

I'm not the only one working to fill in gaps. Disabled artists and activists have been pushing for years to get the mainstream to understand the importance of authentic depictions of disability that are created, shaped, and portrayed by actual disabled people.

Finally, in the past few years, multiple projects featuring authentic depictions of disability, such as the documentary *Crip Camp*[3] and the Netflix series *Special*,[4] have broken through into the mainstream. Meanwhile, in nerd culture, important works like the anthology *Disabled People Destroy Science Fiction*[5] and the *Fate Accessibility*

Toolkit[6]—resources created by impressive teams of contributors—point the way to a more inclusive and accessible future.

Super Sick: Making Peace with Chronic Illness is an important contribution to this small, but growing, number of resources—providing an authentic voice for the often overlooked experience of chronic illness. Here, Allison Alexander combines her personal experiences with first-hand accounts from other chronically ill people and interweaves them with stories from pop culture. By claiming and finding meaning in these, often imperfect, mainstream stories, Allison carves out space for identities that have spent too long being hidden and silenced.

There are so many things about disability, and chronic illness in particular, that aren't widely understood. Many non-disabled people don't understand that their experiences are different from those of disabled and chronically ill people. For example, having an anxiety disorder is different from being worried, stressed, and nervous. People with anxiety disorders have unique experiences, like anxiety triggers, panic attacks, and repetitive mental cycles. Similarly, chronic pain and chronic illness are unique experiences that are different from temporary pain and short-term illness.

In *Super Sick*, Allison's clear, honest, and humourous voice brings the unique experiences of chronic illness to life. While Allison does talk about the ways that being chronically ill are different from not being sick, at the heart of this book is a humanity that we can all identify with. On the deepest level, this book is about the human struggle to come to terms with suffering. It is also about the desire to be recognized as a whole, imperfect, complex human being and the search for connection, love, and meaning.

Chronic illness can be isolating for those who experience it and those who provide support. But knowing you aren't alone helps, and this book breaks through the silence, shame, and toxic messages that keep people isolated. The truth is that we aren't alone. Chronic illness touches all of our lives. While living with it is challenging, we can follow Allison's lead and reach out to others, come to a place of acceptance, and define what is meaningful in our lives.

SUPERHEROES AREN'T SICK

"Pain is an old friend."[1]

— STEPHEN STRANGE, *DOCTOR STRANGE*

*S*uperheroes aren't sick—have you noticed? Wonder Woman doesn't give up on the planet because she's got a migraine. Link doesn't avoid saving Hyrule because every muscle in his body screams at him to lie down. The Doctor doesn't stay in the TARDIS all day because his immune system demands it. Nope, these characters are all healthy and active—key traits to saving the world.

While these characters might be fictional, they matter. They are significant because stories, real or not, are a big part of culture. Stories shape our lives. They tell our children how to act and inform adults about what is normal. We look up to these characters not just because they are entertaining, but because their struggles mirror our own. All stories speak deeply about what it means to be human.

I just wish more stories resonated with my particular life experience. As someone who wrestles with illness and exhaustion almost every day, I struggle to identify with these characters whom I love. I want to be like them. I want to be a hero.

For me, though, heroism doesn't mean punching Thanos in the face; it means doing small deeds for those around me. Volunteering at events, babysitting my godkids, and even doing the dishes are Herculean tasks for me. Often, my body is incapable of those things.

Messages all around me promote good health as something that's expected—billboards showcasing happy, healthy people; online dating sites where people list "active" as a requirement for their ideal partner; college pamphlets that tell me I can do anything. The very nature of our lives is built around the notion of *doing* things. Healthy people can go to work every day, run errands, visit friends, raise children, attend events, and take on personal projects without thinking twice about it.

The idea of being unable to do everyday tasks easily, of staying home and resting for several days because I used up all my energy going grocery shopping, is foreign to many. The *chronic* part of illness is difficult for people to wrap their minds around if they haven't experienced it themselves.

No one likes pain. Most of us do everything we can to avoid it—even carefully brushing our teeth each day to escape that dreaded news from the dentist (and I *still* get cavities! What gives?). When we hear about IV needles and kidney stones and operations and broken limbs, we wince... and for good reason. No one wants to be ill, in pain, or incapacitated. But at least those problems aren't forever. At least there's that horizon of healthiness to look forward to once that limb is healed or that week-long flu is over.

What if that wound never heals and continues to throb, forever? What if I'm consistently nauseated and bed-ridden? What if I'm always drained of energy—not just the "I'm tired because I didn't get enough sleep" kind of drained, but the "I can barely find the energy to lift a spoon" kind of drained? What if I'm sick for days and days on end, with no healthy future to look forward to because I have a chronic illness? What if "healthy" isn't an option?

THE INCURABLE CLUB

I can be put out of commission at a moment's notice—sent racing to the nearest bathroom with debilitating stomach cramps as though an invisible hand is crushing my gut. These attacks are anywhere between a one and a ten on the pain scale (one being mild discomfort and ten being the apocalypse). They can last anywhere between five minutes and a few hours. They're exhausting, and I never know when they're going to happen. When they're really bad, my body overheats and sometimes I get so woozy with pain that I pass out. After the pain diminishes, I get chills and shakes from aftershock.

I don't look sick—I don't need a wheelchair or a cane, I'm not losing my hair, and I have no visible scars. But I am plagued with this mystery illness.

It's called irritable bowel syndrome, the medical community's elaborate term for "we don't know what's wrong with you or how to fix it."

Since the results of the many tests, pokes, prods, and milkshakes that taste like chalk (a.k.a. barium) came out negative, doctors christened me with this fancy designation, generally referred to as IBS. There are varying degrees of severity, and according to the Mayo Clinic, "Only a small number of people with IBS have severe signs and symptoms."[2] I'm one of that unlucky number. And so are thousands of others, if the online forums and Facebook groups I've participated in are any indication.

My symptoms include those random attacks of abdominal pain and cramping, alternating bouts of diarrhea and constipation, and fatigue. I also have several other issues that may or may not be related, such as iron and B12 deficiency, nausea, insomnia, recurring infections, anxiety, and depression. During the past couple years, I've added chronic pelvic and neck pain to that list.

These problems may be manageable for a short time. But when they keep happening, when there's no bright horizon of "getting better" to look forward to, I feel like I'm a cup continually being poured out and never refilled.

Pain is an old friend. But she's the exhausting, I-wish-you-would-leave-already type of friend. She's the kind of friend who barges in on you just as you're heading to an important meeting and makes you late. She kicks you when you're down, hurts you, and stresses you out even when she's not around. People constantly say what a bad friend she is and that you should cut her out of your life for good, but she persists no matter what you try. I wish I could send her packing, but I'm forced to live with her because I don't have the power to evict her.

There are more illnesses that fall into this mystery category, including lupus, thalassemia, chronic fatigue syndrome/myalgic encephalomyelitis, fibromyalgia, and many others of which I've heard first-hand accounts over the course of writing this book. I am a not-so-proud member of a group—an incurable club.

GROWING UP SICK

I was not particularly athletic or physically strong as a child (those descriptors still apply even now that I'm a grown woman). I had no more willpower than a vampire at a blood drive. And I was certainly not strong enough to deal with my chronic condition. But I didn't have a choice in the matter. I *had* to be strong enough.

I had to persevere and continue living, even when I didn't think I could withstand a second more of agony. When I'd reached my pain threshold, I was pushed past what I thought I could endure. When I reached my emotional limit, I cried and carried on. I didn't talk about my illness much; it was simply the part of my life I tried to ignore until it slapped me in the face.

I remember getting up extra early on school days so I would have time to sit on the toilet for half an hour before catching the bus; I always got cramps in the morning before school, because stress can trigger IBS, and I was always stressed. I remember the anxiety it caused, never knowing when or where I would be when the pain hit again, but always knowing it was coming to find me. I remember sitting in class, experiencing cramps and hot flashes but trying to wait it out until recess because it was embarrassing asking to go to the bathroom so often.

My life looked so different from my friends' lives, though most of them had no idea what I was going through. They would gush excitedly about an upcoming class trip while I agonized over whether or not to go. Sometimes the stress and fear of having a sudden attack nowhere near a bathroom just wasn't worth it. I had most of the same worries they did—school, friends, crushes, acne, family, popularity, future… with the additions of chronic pain, exhaustion, depression, fear, and self-consciousness due to illness. I envied my healthy friends for the freedom they had.

When I was house-sitting for family friends, I had friends over to hang out. One of the girls came out of the bathroom and criticized the rack of magazines by the toilet.

"Who needs to read in the bathroom? You're in there for, like, one minute," she scoffed.

I remember laughing and nodding along with everyone else. Except, I had a stack of comics on a rack in my bathroom at home, and a book tucked in the cabinet below the sink. I carried one in my purse when I went out. I appreciated it when people in homes I visited kept books in their bathrooms because then I had something to read in case I had an attack there and didn't have time to grab my purse (or felt awkward doing so). I've been on the toilet for up to four hours in intense pain, and reading sometimes helps as a distraction. But I was too embarrassed to speak up or mention my lengthy bathroom visits. The cool girl of the group said books didn't belong in the bathroom, so I pretended to agree.

I didn't talk much about my illness. I thought it was shameful. Few people knew about my condition besides my parents and my teachers (whom my mom informed in case I needed to leave class quickly to visit the bathroom).

The only people I felt understood my illness were my mom and one of her friends (an honourary aunt), who both had IBS as well. I was thankful for their presence in my life, but there was no one my own age to relate to. Or if there was, they were also tight-lipped about it.

In high school, I went on a week-long class trip to Chicago, and one of our stops was the Six Flags amusement park. One of my most vivid memories from that trip is having an IBS attack in the morning. I was in the hotel bathroom while my entire class, plus chaperones, waited in a running bus for me. FYI: knowing people are waiting on you does not reduce the stress of being sick. I bet none of my classmates even thought about the incident again after the bus started moving, but I remember the embarrassment and the pain. I was unable to go on any of the roller coasters that day because the after-effects of the attack left me drained and unable to do much. I felt depressed wandering around the theme park, weak and unable to ride the roller coasters.

University is mostly a fuzzy, unpleasant memory because I spent the majority of it holed up by myself. I'm already an introvert, but being sick didn't help my socialization habits. I had been trying a special diet for IBS, which at first seemed to help, but then made things worse. I attended class, went back to my on-campus apartment, was sick, did my work, and went to bed: rinse and repeat. While my friends were attending parties, running social justice campaigns, cheering on sports teams, and texting me about their latest crushes, I was literally sick to my stomach—not over their wonderfully stereotypical college lives, but over the chronic disease I wish I had left behind with my high school woes.

I made friends with the girls in the apartment next to mine, and they kept me from becoming a complete hermit, but I often traded friendship for exhaustion. Never mind boyfriends and barbecues—I barely had the energy to stop by the grocery store to stock my empty fridge. My Friday nights consisted, primarily, of curling up on a couch in front of *Buffy the Vampire Slayer* with a pillow and a blanket. There was something about seeing a teenager slaying demons that gave me comfort in facing my own medical monsters.

After graduating, I faced a new challenge: finding work. After months of searching, I landed a nine-to-five office job working in advertising and design at a newspaper.

At first, my bosses were sympathetic when I took sick days, but they became less understanding and more annoyed as my leaves of absence added up. Even after explaining I experienced chronic stomach pain, I got anxious thinking they'd assume I was missing work on purpose. I'm a perfectionist who likes to exceed expectations and I hate disappointing people. Despite the fact that I was great at my job, I was failing at attendance. I felt broken and worthless.

FEELING WORTHLESS

I struggled to accept that I had limits. I felt other people were more valuable than I was. All the messages society sent me confirmed my fears, declaring that I deserved health, wealth, and happiness. If I didn't embody those things, I was not getting my due out of life.

If I didn't deny or ignore my illness, I felt relegated to

the sidelines or written off. Sometimes I wrote myself off, unable to feel valued because I couldn't impact the world around me in the ways I wanted. Why should I be loved when there were enough perfectly healthy people to go around? Why should I be considered as valuable as someone who could make it to their job every day? Why should I treat myself with respect when my body constantly betrayed me?

"Living to fight another day is sometimes the most heroic thing you can do," says Elisabeth, a thirty-nine-year-old freelance editor who suffers from connective tissue disorder, ulcerative colitis, and Gilbert's disease. Elisabeth has never been totally well, so she hasn't experienced the shocking loss that some people with chronic illness go through:

"It's been more little things—accepting that I sometimes need a cane, accepting that I do better with a wheelchair when there's a lot of walking involved, accepting that I need to be cautious about food, etc. You just *deal*."

I don't want to be weak. I don't want to be worthless because of an issue I can't control. I don't want to be pushed to the sidelines of my own story because I'm sick. I want to be Thor so I can do what I want, when I want, and make my ancestors proud!

smashes cup on the floor with gusto

But this is not my fate. I am not a nearly indestructible superhero. I am merely human, and a broken one at that.

kneels down to pick up smashed pieces of cup

Though I might not have anything in common with the god of thunder, I have discovered a superhero I *can* relate to: the time-travelling sorcerer from the Marvel universe, Stephen Strange. Doctor Strange understands pain in a way other characters do not, so maybe not *all* heroes are pain-free after all. Strange deals with feelings of frustration and worthlessness after his hands are damaged in a car accident. As a neurosurgeon, his career is all that matters to him. He's set aside friends, relationships, and hobbies in order to become a success, and he can't imagine life without it:

> **Christine:** Some things just can't be fixed.
> **Stephen:** Life without my work…
> **Christine:** Is still life. This isn't the end. There are other things that can give your life meaning.
> **Stephen:** Like what? Like you?

When I first saw *Doctor Strange* in theatres, I remember the audience gasping at this line. Strange's words are selfish and awful, implying not even love is worth his time. He lashes out at the one person who cares about him, pushing her away. And yet his initial reaction— wanting life back to the way it was—is horribly familiar to me; I wish life would revert to a pain-free time, even though I don't remember what that time was like. I wish I could take back every time I pushed someone away because of the pain.

Stephen Strange defines himself by his job, and when that's gone, he doesn't know what to do with himself. He's angry and in denial—well-known emotions for those who suffer. "I'm not getting any better!" he shouts at Christine, and I shout with him. I know how he feels. Losing your health can feel like losing your life. There is often no going back, and for those of us who've been sick since we can remember, there's no back to return to in the first place.

THE WARM HUG OF SELF-PITY

It's easy to feel sorry for yourself when you're in pain all the time. I experience sadness, anger, grief, bitterness, and ALL THE EMOTIONS. I retreat into my misery, certain no one else can understand. I'm not even sure I want anyone to understand, not really, because that would mean letting someone in and letting myself feel a smidgen of comfort, or even hope. And that's not what my pain is about. It's about me. It's about *my* suffering. And everyone else should stay away and feel sorry for me!

That's Doctor Strange's attitude too, and look how well it works out for him: he sits alone in his million-dollar home, spurning the company of the one person who cares about him, wearing his misery like a cloak that wraps around him with a mind of its own. He doesn't just search for a solution to his disability—he demands it, obstinately chasing after anything that might result in a cure. And he doesn't just want his hands healed, he wants them back the way they were so he can perform surgery again. He pushes aside any alternate solutions to his problem, such as Christine's suggestion of finding new things to value in life. He wallows in self-pity.

Stephen Strange is a jerk-face. I understand *why* he's a jerk-face, but that doesn't make him any less of a jerk. I don't want to end up like him, but the temptation to wrap myself in self-pity's warm hug is there.

Self-pity chokes relationships and drains joy, becoming a comfortable default setting even though it's unhealthy. But the other option is more difficult. As Doctor Strange discovers, it requires admitting you're imperfect, that you have to face a new sort of life—one that includes brokenness.

The tendency to pity myself is partly rooted in a society that's constantly telling me I deserve better, but also in my own desire to be loved and accepted. Self-pity is self-centred and doesn't leave room for real relationships.

At first, when I tried to address this behaviour in myself, I thought I had to squash down all the emotions I was going through. All that did was add guilt into the mix. Pain, frustration, anger, bitterness, *and* guilt—it's not a happy combo. But then I realized feeling these emotions is okay; it's the way I react to them that matters. I don't have to be a jerk-face even if I feel like being one.

I don't plaster a smile on my face when I'm suffering. I'm still disheartened. I still sob when I don't think I can handle any more pain. But I'm not like Doctor Strange at the beginning of his movie, when he pushes away everyone who cares about him. Because I've found it's those people who make life worth living.

Loneliness aggravates self-pity, and spending time with others helps me have a more balanced perspective. Laughing, focusing on something other than myself, and finding quiet times for prayer or solace helps me remember where my value comes from. Accepting my condition is also important, but it's hard—because who in their right mind wants to accept a life of suffering?

LOSING AGAIN AND AGAIN

It takes Stephen Strange an entire movie to arrive at a point of acceptance, which is just a snapshot of how long the process can take. As an already arrogant person, he struggles to come to terms with his condition, but he can't find peace—he can't move past self-pity and pride—until he acknowledges that his life looks different than others'.

Stephen's maniacal search leads him to the Ancient One, who teaches him what is essentially magic to advance the plot of the movie. Ironically, the advice given to Stephen, "Forget everything you know," applies not just to the manipulating of portals and time, but to the experience of chronic pain as well. Forget everything you know about life, because illness can change it all. Sickness is like Dormammu—the film's villain—an antagonist determined to put heroes through the wringer.

It's difficult to let change, and being different, sink in. Especially if you're like me, because I like what's familiar. To demonstrate the extent that I hate change, consider how I, at ten years old, cried when my family installed new windows in our house. That's right, *windows*. Better, nicer-looking windows that kept the house warmer than the old ones. But they were different. They were new. And I whined at my dad for daring to install them. *Bring back the old windows with the paint chipping off the wood, Dad!*

It was a long road to accepting those new, white, aluminum windows, but maybe now that I've done it, I can tackle accepting my illness.

What I like most about *Doctor Strange* is that the story

doesn't solve all of Stephen's problems through miraculous healing.

Though he approaches the Ancient One to heal his hands, Stephen Strange forgoes that choice so he can be part of something larger: defeating the ruler of the Dark Dimension and learning to be humble. I don't get that choice where my illness is concerned, and I don't know if I'd make the decision to accept my condition were I in his shoes, but I admire him for it.

> **Stephen:** So I could have my hands back again? My old life?
>
> **Ancient One:** You could. And the world would be all the lesser for it.

My illness has shaped my life in ways I didn't ask for or want, but it's significant that I wouldn't be who I am without it. Chronic pain has affected everything from my personality to my job to my community to my religious beliefs. I have stumbled through a number of experiences, emotions, and crises that have made me more equipped to understand others who are in pain, and more driven to search for peace. I'd rather not have gone through the pain, but at least some good has come out of something horrible.

Those of us with chronic pain have something unique to offer, not in spite of our pain, but because of it. It's okay to grieve the losses of chronic illness. It's okay to be broken; everyone is in some way. Just because we're unfixable doesn't mean we're worthless.

At the end of *Doctor Strange*, Stephen faces off against Dormammu—not once or twice, but over and over again.

He traps the evil being in a time loop, withstanding multiple deaths until Dormammu agrees to leave Earth alone.

> **Dormammu:** You will never win.
> **Stephen:** No, but I can lose again and again. And again. Forever.

I like this analogy because it means that I, as a suffering person, can be a warrior like Doctor Strange. Or chronic illness wizard, if you will. Suffering people can find meaning in life just the same. We lose again and again. And again. Forever. But we still choose to fight. If I consider myself this way, I am a superhero instead of a character relegated to the sidelines, even if I don't feel very mighty.

The best superheroes aren't omnipotent, perfect characters; they have flaws, just like I do. They are broken, just like I am. There's strength in that brokenness, and maybe that in itself is my superpower.

2

INVALID: A DIRTY WORD

"Side note: *invalid*. Whoever invented that word, and made it the same word as not-valid? That person sucked."[1]

— AZA RAY, *MAGONIA* BY MARIA DAHVANA HEADLEY

"My history is hospitals." The first line in the fantasy novel *Magonia* instantly grabs my attention. The story is narrated by a teenager named Aza, who is just as messed up as I am. She has a mysterious lung disease that makes her unable to breathe, and no one knows what's wrong with her:

"I try not to get involved with my disease, but it's persuasive. When it gets ahold of me, the gasping can put me on the floor, flopping and whistling, something hauled up from a lake bottom. Sometimes I wish I could go back to the bottom and start over somewhere else. As some*thing* else."

Aza gets it. Sometimes I just want to start over too.

There's this question we sci-fi nerds sometimes ask each other—would you transfer your consciousness into a robotic body if you could? We debate the ethical and practical repercussions. Would I still have a soul without human blood and bones? Would I miss the feeling of human touch? Would I still be me? But when I'm hunched over with cramps, the morality of the question is irrelevant. Sign. Me. Up.

The desire to feel connected to and accepted by others is built into us. We want to feel like we belong, like we are home. Pain separates us from that feeling.

Aza is isolated from the other children in her school because she struggles with something they can't understand. "Secretly, as in only semi-secretly," she narrates, "as in this is a thing I say loudly sometimes—I think I wasn't meant to be human. I don't work right."

Aza respects the people who treat her like a normal human being—the girl at school who makes fun of her, the teacher who puts her in detention for misbehaving, and especially her best friend, Jason—because they don't treat her like a piece of glass that might break if they speak to her. Though she's not suicidal, the thought does cross her mind that the pain—her own physical and emotional pain, as well as the inconvenience she causes to the people around her—would be solved if she didn't exist.

Like Aza, I notice that when I tell people I'm ill, they want to fix me. I once mentioned my condition to an acquaintance and received the reply, "Oh, have you been to the doctor? You should go to the doctor. I hope you feel better soon."

This was a well-intentioned comment made by a caring person, but also an ignorant response fuelled by our culture's misconceptions about wellness. It takes the pressure off the healthy person as they have avoided a potentially awkward conversation. It's like when people ask, "How are you?" and you automatically reply, "I'm fine" no matter what you're feeling.

Suggesting I see a doctor when I've seen enough to last three lifetimes is a discouraging reminder I don't need. Doctors are not Panacea's children, ready to gift their patients with cure-all remedies. And telling me to feel better isn't uplifting, because I'm not likely to get better— that's what *chronic* illness means. Responses like this suggest I'm only acceptable if I'm healed.

I'M STILL SICK

In TV shows, characters often get sick for a single episode and recover by the next. For example, in the *Buffy the Vampire Slayer* episode "Killed by Death," Buffy gets the flu. Her sickness is the catalyst to get her into the hospital so she can solve a mystery involving a demon preying on sick kids. Her illness is relevant because only fevered children can see the monster, but it's also fleeting.

Sometimes a brief illness is used to make one character worry about another, such as in *The Hunger Games* when Peeta gets a fever and Katniss has to find medicine for him. There is something touching about one character caring for the other, especially in a potentially romantic relationship. This is, no doubt, why so many Jane Austen novels include a woman falling ill to the distress of her potential lover—the threat of losing someone to illness can spur a character to admit their feelings.

In many video games, there are standard items that counteract poison or work against specific diseases; it's literally built into these games that status ailments can be cured in a moment and your character is useless until they are. Sometimes, sickness or disability is magically healed instantly (like in the fairy tale "Rapunzel," when the prince's blindness is cured by Rapunzel's tears). Other times, it's treated as a joke. I was watching an episode of *The Office*, and my ears perked up at the mention of irritable bowel syndrome:

> **Michael:** There have been reports around the office that you have been talking baby talk.
> **Andy:** Why would people say that?
> **Michael:** Well, I have it on good authority that you said the following [hands Andy a note card]. Can you read that back to me?
> **Andy:** "Andy have a boo-boo tummy." Would you rather me say, "Hey guys, my Irritable Bowel Syndrome is flaring up. Crazy diarrhea happening right now." 'Cause things could get real adult REAL fast![2]

Andy's irritable bowel is never mentioned again after this scene. Not once. It was brought up as a joke with no hint of the pain this illness can cause, and Andy lives a perfectly normal, healthy life throughout the rest of the show.

I can't help wishing my illness wasn't dismissed so easily. It's fitting that *The Office* is one of two shows I've ever seen reference it, because IBS is one of those awkward-to-mention illnesses and *The Office* is nothing if not wonderfully awkward. The other show is *Parks and Recreation*, which is just as hilariously uncomfortable as *The Office* and, similarly, uses Jeremy Jamm's IBS as the butt of a joke.

Other stories, like movies *A Walk to Remember* and *Love Story*, use sick characters as a plot device to teach healthy people how to live fuller lives. The show *Speechless* pokes fun at this concept by demonstrating that JJ, a sixteen-year-old with cerebral palsy, is a normal kid with as much sass as the next teenager. In the pilot episode, he's greeted with applause from his classmates when he enters his new school for no other reason than being in a wheelchair; he is even recommended for class president.

"Why? You don't know me," he asks through his communication board in response to a "JJ for President" sign being flashed in his face.

"Well, we don't have to. You're an inspiration," a teacher replies.[3]

As ridiculous as this sounds, it's an accurate representation of our culture's common response to people with disabilities, illnesses, and chronic pain; suffering people need to be inspirations for others. If you are not a charismatic go-getter, your job options are limited when you have a disability. JJ can't work as a cashier, do manual labour, or wait tables like many teenagers his age. But his inability to do those things doesn't mean his job is automatically to make others feel better about their own existence. Like JJ, who counteracts these stigmas, *Magonia*'s Aza is ostracized because she refuses to be put into that mould, treating those who don't know how to respond to her with disdain and sarcasm instead of "inspiring" them.

Chronic illness and disability are hard to write around if they aren't the main crux of a story. Hence, we have many stories about cancer patients, but not so many about people who are important characters outside of their illnesses. Audiences want heroes to overcome their challenges, and chronic issues can't be fixed. Many writers think if their story features a character who is chronically ill, that story needs to be *about* that sickness. Because what else is there to say? Once you're the victim of a chronic illness, you're done.

In addition to being featured in storylines that primarily focus on healing, inspiration, or comedy, sick characters are often depicted inaccurately or not included at all. This is disheartening to those of us looking for validation. It's frustrating that this is the cultural norm, because people unwittingly tell me I'm missing out on life when I say, "I'm sick," and they respond, "Again?" It's not that I'm sick *again*, it's that I'm *still* sick. It's not something I can control with the flick of a remote, as much as I wish I could, and an impatient response doesn't help the guilt I feel from cancelling plans for the tenth time.

TOO MANY THINGS GOING ON

People who suffer from chronic illnesses often have more than one condition. Once that first problem hits, it sends your body into a never-ending downward spiral. It would be fair if we spread around all the illnesses among all the healthy people, but nooo, all the sicknesses get funnelled down to the already miserable.

My own long list of issues *might* be related to each other, and I'm sure my compromised immune system impacts things, but they're not all lumped into one diagnosis. The body is a complex piece of machinery that we don't entirely understand, and when one thing goes wrong, other things can follow.

Multiple conditions can increase feelings of worthlessness. I sometimes wonder if people will stop believing me when I tell them my latest issue. If I don't present a doctor's note with a specific diagnosis every time, will they start to think I'm making these things up to get attention? How many health problems will be allowed until it's one too many, the final straw before they get tired of hearing about my issues?

When chronic illness gets piled on with *other* life events or factors, it's also a recipe for stress. For me, life events that are already difficult—moving to a new place, changing jobs, arguing with a friend or family member, grieving a lost loved one, feeling helpless while a friend grieves, feeling stigmatized because of illness or gender—can trigger my IBS, but they are unavoidable. (For example, I experience extra stress in the doctor's office because I'm a woman, a common occurrence for sick women that I'll go into more detail later.)

Being part of several minorities at once can weigh you down further when you add it to an illness. There are stigmas that exist in the medical community, whether you're a woman, a person of colour, a non-binary gender, etc.

"Sometimes it can just feel like I have too many special

things going on," says Niko, a non-binary transmasculine twenty-five-year-old with Ehlers-Danlos syndrome. "For example, talking to professors about medical accommodations and pronouns. Illness can also make things complicated—for example, I can't bind easily due to unstable ribs. Shopping for affirming clothes is further limited by the braces and orthotics I wear daily. And there is also a component of feeling like being sick itself is a feminine thing, and that being seen as a delicate fragile man would be a lot worse than where I am now."

Niko is facing stigmas from multiple places—from the fact that they are trans, from being sick, from showing visible signs of disability through braces and orthotics, and from their own fear and experience of being sick as a feminine issue. Plus, doctors aren't necessarily trained in how to properly treat LGBTQ2 patients and may write off symptoms.

"The doctor didn't seem to know much about sex between women—and the fact that women can still get STIs from unsafe sex with female partners. Or, if he did know, he didn't speak up," writes Caroline Praderio in an *Insider* article as she relates the experience of a lesbian patient.[4]

Chronic illness makes every stressor heavier, whether it's related to gender, relationships, family, finances, work, addiction, or something else. Many don't feel they have the strength to face so many issues and stigmas at once. It takes courage, community, and patience to stand up for yourself.

FRIENDS MAY SAY THE WRONG THING

North America is steeped in diet and fitness culture, which idealizes health in many ways and demands people look a certain way. Be thin. Be fit. Be healthy. Those are the messages stemming from most visual media, with actors who fall into a specific category of beauty and models who are airbrushed and photoshopped in pre-production. These are damaging ideals, even for those who do not struggle with chronic illnesses. While there's nothing wrong with exercising and eating healthy foods, the country's obsession with youth, health, and beauty has created a culture of body shaming and impossible standards. It's further perpetuated by diet companies; because they know that people will spend money on their products, diet, gain the weight back, and "need" the products again, they promote diet culture to make money.

There are also growing movements toward natural health care—promoting special diets, organic foods, natural supplements, etc. I've seen social media posts from multi-level marketing promoters about how much their lives have changed since they started using [insert supplement here]. With hashtags like #microbiome and #naturalhealth, they post about how they used to be a depressed, unhealthy lump just like me and now their world is filled with rainbows and butterflies. Wouldn't I like to attain their level of healthiness? Wouldn't I like to mirror the photo of them standing on the beach in Hawaii with their hands lifted to the glorious sunrise in praise? All it would take is $200 a month for a supplement that is not FDA approved and runs the risk of making my symptoms worse, not better.

I get frustrated by these messages, because they imply I could be happy too if I just put in some effort. As if I'm not trying. As if I haven't tried. As if I *want* to be sick.

I don't disapprove of testing cures for your body's problems. I'm not against trying specific foods, supplements, or lifestyle changes to improve health; for example, I've gone to a dietician, I try to eat healthy, and I use peppermint oil for bowel spasms and allergies. My problem is not with people trying to feel better or even with people selling products that they believe in. It's when those people judge me because I'm not better. It's when people assume what has worked for them will automatically work for someone else. And it's when people equate bad health with a meaningless life.

SOMETIMES, I browse drugstores to examine the messages in get-well cards. I got the idea from Philip Yancey, who mentions in his book *Where Is God When It Hurts?* that all the messages in these cards are about getting well as fast as possible. They suggest you're "missing out" on life until you're better.

Yancey made this observation in 1977, and not much has changed since then. In my own perusal, I read a card that said, "While You're in the Hospital, hope that each day brings something happy—sunshine through your window, friendly smiles, some pleasant news… whatever will make the time pass quickly until you feel better again."

Another card features an adorable dog on the cover and says, "Heal!!" followed by "a.k.a. feel better soon" and a Bible verse: "I pray that you may enjoy good health and that all may go well with you" (3 John 1:2, NIV). The inclusion of this verse makes me especially uncomfortable. The author of this card used a book I value to promote an ideal that not all of us can aspire to.

These cards are designed with temporary illnesses in mind, of course. But they do suggest life can't properly go on until you're better. Even the title of the subsection in the greeting card aisle, "Get-Well Cards," points toward health as a necessary commodity.

I'm just as guilty as the next person of idealizing healthiness just like these cards do. "Hope you feel better soon" is my automatic response when someone tells me they're sick. What else are you supposed to say? It's not like I want them to stay sick. I have trouble coming up with an alternate response and sometimes there just isn't a "right" thing to say.

I stumbled across a website that sells greeting cards, but there is no "Get-Well" section. Instead, along with the usual "Birthday," "Anniversary," and "Thank You" categories, there's a tab for "Empathy." The business was created by Emily McDowell, who writes on her blog:

> "Most of us struggle to find the right words in the face of a friend or loved one's major health crisis, whether it's cancer, chronic illness, or mental illness, or anything else... we don't have the right language for it. 'Get well soon' cards don't make sense when someone might not."[5]

Emily, who is a cancer survivor, intimately understands the isolation that can occur when family and friends disappear because they don't know what to say.

After a quick scroll-through, I was immediately a fan of these empathy cards. "How about this," one of the cards reads, "The next non-doctor who thinks they can cure you gets smothered with kale." Another says, "Well, this just sucks. I wish I had a better way to say it, but my brain feels totally stuck right now. But I just want you to know that even though I might not always have exactly the right words, you will always have me. I'm not going anywhere. So I hope you're cool with that. Because I love you." And a third says, "You're not a burden. You're a human."

These cards hit empathy on the nose, and they capture what my friends and family are trying to say when they tell me, "Get better soon."

A few months into our relationship, my boyfriend was doing an amazing job adjusting to dating someone with a chronic illness. He didn't mind when I cancelled on him or if we stayed in because I was too exhausted to leave the house. He would message me the next day, asking if I was feeling better. His questions came out of love—he didn't want me to be in pain. But I experienced this uncomfortable feeling of uncertainty, questioning my value every time he asked and I was *not* feeling better. "Yes" was the easy answer, even if it wasn't true; it was the expected answer. Saying, "No, I still feel like crap," is such a downer.

I didn't speak up about my feelings at first because I knew he meant well. But eventually, I asked, "But it's okay if I'm not better, right? If I *never* get better, are you going to be all right with it?" I explained that I didn't mind if he asked how I was feeling, but it would help me emotionally if he clarified that he still cared about me even if I wasn't better.

"Of *course* it's fine if you're not better—I care about you no matter what!" he said immediately, a little horrified that his words—a seemingly innocent question—had affected me negatively. Despite the fact that I *knew* he accepted me, it was a relief to hear him say it in the context of my illness; there was this little nugget of fear in me that wondered if he was waiting for my health to improve and would give up on me if it didn't.

After that conversation, he started rephrasing his queries. He would ask me, "How are you feeling today?" instead of, "Are you feeling better?"—which turned a loaded question into a totally manageable one. I also appreciated the addition of "today" or "right now," because it acknowledged the fickleness of my health— good one minute and bad the next—and reminded me I can take life one day, one hour, one minute at a time.

FRIENDS MAY SAY THE REALLY WRONG THING

One of the worst things someone can accuse me of is lying about or faking my illness. Whether it's a doctor who can't figure out what's wrong and believes I'm making it up, a friend who suspects I just want attention, or a boss who thinks I'm skipping work on purpose, this type of response stings like Bilbo's Elven blade.

I am surrounded by friends who are incredibly understanding, and for that I am thankful. But there are people in my life who don't get it, who don't comprehend that by texting jokingly, "Oh, you're sick again. Suuure," as if I'm making it up, they are cutting into my self-esteem. And there will always be people like that.

There will never be a universal understanding of

chronic pain unless everyone experiences it, which isn't going to happen. Many don't even know this kind of life needs to be acknowledged in the first place.

Hannah, a thirty-year-old writer who suffers from epilepsy, sometimes wakes up on the floor because her heart literally stops and she falls over. She's dealt with missing vision, slower processing, short-term memory loss, and trouble remembering words she knows how to use (aphasia).

When a friend told her she believed Hannah's seizures were all in her mind and she was faking it, Hannah was crushed.

"For someone to accuse me of that, even if it was a mistake, is ripping," Hannah says. "No one wants to fake this. It's not like you want days off. I don't enjoy being in the hospital for eight hours. I don't enjoy calling the ambulance for myself.

"A lot of people, when I tell them about aphasia, are like, 'Oh, that happens to me all the time.' And I'm like, no… Sure, these things have happened to you occasionally because the brain is faulty. But this happens to me a lot, and it affects my self-esteem. I have a big vocabulary that I often can't access."

Comparing her condition to forgetting that one word on the tip of your tongue is like comparing a golf ball to the Death Star. It's not the same thing.

Empathy is not possible, or required, from everyone around us, though it *is* an incredibly validating experience. I appreciate that my adulthood best friend also has IBS (though I don't wish it on him or anyone). He makes me feel at ease and is one of the few people I enjoy travelling with because, if I spend twenty minutes too long in the bathroom, he knows, without asking, what's up. If I make us late for whatever event we've travelled to because I need to sleep off the pain first, he understands. If I'm anxious, he knows why.

There is a sense of affirmation that comes from knowing you're not alone, and that simple fact can bring peace through turmoil.

However, though empathy is wonderful, I don't discount the people who want to make a compassionate space for my pain even if they have never experienced it themselves. Often, sick people don't have the energy to take care of each other, and it's the healthy people who are able to step up. I have other friends and family who are incredibly compassionate people despite the fact that they've never experienced chronic pain.

Sometimes I'm so battered by misconceptions that I don't bother trying to explain to those who want to understand. Yet if I keep trying, I'll eventually find those few people who make me feel safe and are willing to make a space in their lives for me and my illness.

HAVE YOU TRIED NOT BEING SICK?

"At school, the whole rare-disease-impending-doom situation makes me freakishly intriguing," Aza narrates in *Magonia*. "In the real world, it makes me a problem. Worried look, bang, nervous face, bang: 'Maybe you should talk to someone about your feelings, Aza,' along with a nasty side dish of what-about-God-what-about-therapy-what-about-antidepressants? Sometimes also what-about-faith-healers-what-about-herbs-what-about-crystals-what-about-yoga? Have you tried yoga, Aza, I mean have you, because it helped this friend of a friend who was supposedly dying but didn't, due to downward dog?"

The people who give advice often mean well. But when that conversation is not tempered by a close relationship, it suggests I'm unacceptable the way I am. I'm tempted to yell at the random strangers who give unsolicited advice because they just don't get it. Here are some common responses I've received when someone hears I'm sick:

- Why haven't you been to the doctor?
- You should exercise more.
- Are you getting enough sleep?
- You don't look sick.
- You should try [insert advice here]. My friend tried it and it worked.
- Things could be worse.
- Are you still sick?
- I wish *I* didn't have to go to work/school.
- Your body just needs deliverance; let me pray for you. Didn't work? Let me pray harder.
- Here's some unsolicited diet advice.
- Yeah, I'm tired too.
- You're cancelling again?
- God never gives us more than we can handle.
- Things will get better.

It would almost be easier to ignore if people were callous on purpose. Instead, the problem is misunderstanding, which, in a way, is much harder to deal with. It invalidates my pain when strangers give unsolicited advice as if they're the authority on this thing and if I followed their suggestions I'd be fine.

While I know people like solving problems and feeling useful, sometimes the most helpful response is, "I can't imagine what that's like, but that must be hard." Or send me one of those cards from Emily McDowell, because she knows "When life gives you lemons, I won't tell you a story about my cousin's friend who died of lemons." Or don't say anything at all, because sometimes there just isn't anything to say, and that's okay.

3

DOCTOR HOUSE KNOWS BEST.
SOMETIMES. MAYBE.

"Life is pain! I wake up every morning, I'm in pain! I go to work in pain! Do you know how many times I wanted to just give up?!"[1]

— GREGORY HOUSE, *HOUSE*

*W*hen I'm in pain, my first instinct is to find out why. *Oh, my arm hurts. Why does it hurt? Let me pull up my sleeve and AGGHH I'M BLEEDING!* You get the idea. So barring any form of denial, when the pain is internal, the doctor's office is the first step to diagnosis. Modern medicine can give hope. Maybe there's a pill, treatment, exercise, or diet that will make me feel better.

But then again, maybe there's not. Not every illness has a cure. Or if it does, it may take a while to be diagnosed and find something that works.

DOCTORS AND DIAGNOSES

I want my doctor to tell me exactly what's wrong with me and how to fix it, but sometimes all she can do is run more tests. Life isn't an episode of *House*, where the solution is discovered in forty-five minutes and the patient goes home cured. Diagnosis is often a long, horrendous process. And even professionals get it wrong.

It's frustrating to know something terribly wrong is going on with your body but you're unable to name the problem, much less the solution. It's even more frustrating when your pain is invalidated.

After my appendix ruptured when I was ten years old, the doctor took it out and drained the infectious materials in my abdomen, but something still wasn't right.

I couldn't eat without puking. I couldn't move without raging pain in my belly. Simply turning onto my side was agony. I remember having to sleep on my back and being uncomfortable because I'm a side sleeper. And don't get me started on how torturous peeing was; you'd think I'd swallowed knives instead of water.

When my mom told the doctor my symptoms, he glanced at my scrawny form lying in the hospital bed and then scoffed at her. "I'm sure she's fine," he said. "She's just whining to get attention."

Um, excuse me? Peeing knives over here.

"No, she's not!" my typically non-confrontational mother replied. "She doesn't usually complain at all! Something's wrong."

My mom was right. There were complications that led to me staying in the hospital for weeks after my appendix surgery. The doctor had made an assumption. He didn't know me or understand that I was fairly accustomed to pain.

I can see how someone who interacts with people in pain every day could become indifferent or cynical. It must be hard to retain empathy, or even sympathy, when hearing health complaints is your day-to-day.

The fact that I'm not a complainer is, actually, one of the reasons my appendix ruptured before my parents took me to the hospital. Well, that and because my cousin had just been sick with a terrible flu. His parents had actually taken him to the hospital because they thought *he* had appendicitis, and it turned out he didn't. So I can't blame my parents for thinking I had caught his germs. They didn't realize just how much pain I was in until I started convulsing, and by then it was too late. *Kapow. Splurch.* Those are the sounds an appendix makes when it explodes. True story.

Having a high pain tolerance does not mean I feel pain less than anyone else; it just means I don't show it as much as others. Unfortunately, this stoicism is detrimental when you're in an emergency room and talking coherently to a nurse about how much pain you're in. They tend to place you lower on the priority list.

"I've seen people who have a terrible condition, like a perforated bowel, and should be screaming in pain because it's a terrible infection raging in their stomach, and they are just sitting there chatting with you," says John Neufeld, an emergency doctor in Winnipeg, Manitoba. "And you see the opposite, too, like someone who has nicked their finger and is literally screaming at you about it."

John mentions that because pain is subjective, you

have to take a patient's word for it. But doctors also keep their eyes out for patients who may have ulterior motives or have a history of being cut off of medication. It's a tough position to be in because some people have extremely high pain thresholds and others do not.

There's only so much a doctor can do for chronic pain. John mentions that doctors basically have four options for pain control: analgesics (like Tylenol), anti-inflammatories (like Advil), opiates (like fentanyl), and neuropathic pain medications (like amitriptyline). None of these methods is great for chronic pain. Analgesics often don't help; anti-inflammatories can damage kidneys and cause gastrointestinal bleeding; opiates are addictive and can have other complications as you gain a tolerance for them and require more; neuropathic medications often cause side effects and don't provide pain relief. All of these meds are what doctors refer to as a "high number to treat," which means they only work for a few people out of a large sample size. In other words, even if you can withstand the side effects, it's unlikely the medication will help at all.

"By definition, if you have chronic pain, it's one of two things," John says. "Either 1) we don't know what's wrong, or 2) there's no effective way to manage what's wrong. Family doctors often don't phrase it this way to patients, because they don't want to take away hope."

John says he will often be forthright with his patients and tell them that the medical community doesn't have a good understanding of what causes their pain: "Until we get a better understanding or more studies come out or we develop a new test, you're kind of stuck with the pain that you have." Sometimes, if he knows the patient and their background, he will even tell them it's unlikely they will be rid of their pain. "This helps give them a more accurate picture of their pain management and helps them learn to cope with it as opposed to constantly searching for the next thing that will magically fix a problem that we don't really understand," he says.

I appreciate this type of honesty from medical professionals. It doesn't mean there isn't hope. "To me, hope is independent of the statistical probability that you will find a clear, magical fix," John says. "For me, hope comes from the idea that no matter how shitty things are, there are always things you can do to cope with your situation and develop better strategies for dealing with the situation that you're in, as opposed to dreaming of a solution. It's realistic hope as opposed to unrealistic hope."

A DOCTOR'S SYMPATHY

Not every doctor is good at bedside manner. John mentions he tries to communicate that he cares, that he wishes the patient wasn't in pain, and that he is doing everything in his power to decrease their pain, but doctors can only go so far with sympathy. I certainly don't expect, or want, doctors to break into tears in front of me after hearing about my pain. But I do want them to validate it.

The words of medical professionals hold weight. Doctors have gone through years of study, schooling, and practice to get where they are. They are far more qualified to diagnose an illness than I am. However, they are not qualified to tell me that I must not be in that much pain or that the pain I'm feeling isn't real simply because they can't determine its origin.

Doctor House (from the TV show *House)* would disagree with me. "Everybody lies," he says, a sentence that becomes a mantra in the show. Each episode of *House* is built around this idea of secret-keeping; part of the show's mystery is what the patient isn't telling House's team, and it's a thrill when they discover the truth. Deception is one of the reasons House doesn't bother meeting his patients in person. He assumes that they will lie to him about something crucial and that looking at X-rays and other test results will give him all the information he needs to diagnose their problems.

I can't begin to explain how offensive this attitude is and what the accusation of lying can do to a person suffering from chronic pain. It makes for a fascinating TV show, but in reality, a doctor with House's attitude can cause psychological damage to a patient who genuinely needs help.

Being accused of lying when I'm telling the truth invokes deep, gut-wrenching frustration. And when the accusation is from a medical professional, this frustration is a hundred times worse. For one thing, my physical health is on the line; if my doctor doesn't believe me, how am I supposed to get help for my pain? For another, my mental health is on the line; if my doctor does not confirm my pain, why would others believe me when I tell them? Even friends and family are likely to question my word compared to a doctor's.

In an online article titled "Where is chronic illness represented in popular culture?" writer Naomi Chainey recalls watching an episode of *House* where a patient is diagnosed with chronic fatigue syndrome, the same condition Naomi struggles with.

"House gave the man a long-suffering eyebrow, filled a pill bottle with candy, and presented it as a cure. Hilarious!" she writes. "I cried that night. The disabling illness that had taken my career, my independence and my social life had just been trivialized to viewers the world over, and the worst of it was, I knew there would be no outcry. Too few people knew enough to care."[2]

That episode of *House* even revisits the joke at the end —the patient who had complained of chronic fatigue returns to the hospital asking the staff for a refill of his "prescription." House smiles sarcastically at his coworker, asking, "Got change for a dollar?" so he can refill the pill bottle with candy.[3]

Ha. Ha. Ha. While I am a fan of sarcasm (partly why I enjoy watching *House* in the first place), is House right to be so cynical about people's motives and conditions?

It's true that people lie, sometimes unintentionally. But I'd like the benefit of the doubt. More than that, I want validation from my doctor, my peers, and society. Yes, I am in pain. There might not be a name for my disease, but that doesn't mean my suffering isn't real. House dismisses the mental support that could encourage patients to find hope through their suffering.

In a textbook for nursing students, Pamela D. Larsen writes, "When a diagnosis is finally made, the [patient] frequently shows a somewhat joyous initial response to having a name for the recurrent and troublesome symptoms. This reaction results from the decrease in stress over the unknown.... They seek to achieve the legitimacy necessary to elicit sympathy and avoid stigma, and to protect their own self-concept."[4]

Roughly translated, we're relieved that we're not crazy. I mean, I know I'm not crazy, but it's nice to have someone else confirm that. Advocating for myself gets tiring, and putting a name to an illness legitimizes it. Being diagnosed also means maybe, just maybe, there's hope I won't be in pain forever. Maybe there's research being done on the condition. Maybe there are other people suffering from the same thing—and even if they haven't found a cure, at least I'm not alone.

MEDICATIONS AND SIDE EFFECTS

While many viewers laugh at House's crotchety, cruel behaviour because it seems overblown, I can guess at the source of his attitude. Much like Stephen Strange, House lashes out at those close to him, treating people with derogatory humour and disdain. Unlike the red-cloaked wizard, however, House doesn't receive magic powers or the weight of the universe on his shoulders as a distraction from the pain. House struggles with finding peace, humility, and lasting relationships. He relies on Vicodin to relieve the constant pain in his leg (caused by a golfing accident and ensuing surgery after muscle death). The agony is a constant presence he can never completely get rid of, but the narcotic helps him function.

In another episode of *House*, "Detox," House's boss, Lisa Cuddy, challenges him to go off of Vicodin to prove that he's not addicted to it. Going off the medication incites symptoms of withdrawal and pain, making it impossible for him to do his job. In the end, he admits that he's addicted, and his friends shake their heads sadly at his refusal to stop taking the narcotic.

I'm perplexed by their reaction, as House isn't taking Vicodin because he likes it. He's taking it because it eases his pain. The addiction is real, but it's a side effect of pain management, something that doctors and patients weigh the pros and cons of together when they start treatments. House does go on to abuse this medication and get high from it, which I definitely don't condone. However, I understand why he wants the pain gone.

I wish medications were often as simple as "take this pill, and it will fix your problem." However, even when a medication does address a problem, it often causes a handful of others. When you fill your prescription at the drugstore, it comes with this handy, double-sided, multi-page document that includes all the risks and side effects of taking the treatment.

Here is a list of possible side effects from my latest prescription, a drug to treat nausea:

- diarrhea
- dizziness
- headache
- itchiness
- rash
- abnormal or fast heartbeat
- a fracture
- jitteriness
- nausea or vomiting (ironically)
- sore muscles
- spasms of the hands and feet
- spasm of the voice box

And this is for *one* medication. Like many people with chronic illnesses, I take several—some I take regularly and others on an as-needed basis. I have packages of old prescriptions I never finished because the side effects were too painful, but I keep them around just in case I want to try them again. I have bottles of new prescriptions that I'm trying out to see if they help my condition or not. Then I have a collection of medications for "normal" illnesses—flus, colds, coughs, and allergies—because I never want to be unprepared for those in case I don't have the energy to go to the store. This all comprises an embarrassingly large collection of bottles and packages and medications in my cupboard, which I refer to as my personal pharmacy. I even own one of those weekly pill containers that reminds you what medications to take on what day—the kind normally marketed at the elderly.

When I experience side effects, I have to decide if the treatment is worth it. I've taken a medication that helped me experience fewer attacks of stomach pain, *but* it also gave me perpetual symptoms of a bladder infection. Hmm... stomach pain or bladder infection? Bladder infection or stomach pain? WHY am I choosing between two rotten things? Why can't the question be cake or pie? (The answer to that is easy: pie. Obviously.)

In another episode of *House*, "The Softer Side," House shows up to work happy. That's right, he's downright tickled to be at his job, and everyone's confused by his pleasant behaviour. It turns out he's started taking methadone, and it completely eradicates his pain, though it also slows his breathing to dangerous levels when he sleeps—a side effect he hires someone to keep an eye on.

On this drug, House is friendlier. He's patient with

others. His personality is much improved. But he makes a mistake on the job, letting a patient's parents have their way when he knows better, and blames the methadone: "I screwed up... I played nice because I was in a good mood because it didn't hurt."[5]

House is unwilling to exchange a lack of pain for his sharp intellect—a trade I'd probably be willing to make if I were in his shoes. But his situation brings up another cause and effect that many don't consider: the side effects of pain itself.

It's hard to understand what being in constant pain does to you if you have never experienced it yourself. It's not the same as experiencing a broken arm or getting the flu—there's an end to those things. When the illness is continuous, it's exhausting. When the pain is never ending, regardless of the pain's source, it can even affect your mind and personality.

PAIN AND PERSONALITY

My dad started getting horrible headaches when I was a teenager. They were so bad that he had to take medical leave from work and spent the majority of three years in a dark bedroom just trying to exist through the pain. I didn't see him very often during that time. Occasionally there would be a lull in the headaches, and he'd emerge for a short while, but would retreat soon after. Doctors couldn't figure out what was wrong and pain relievers had no effect. He saw many specialists and had several operations, including the removal of a vein on the side of his head. He had CAT scans and MRIs, but doctors remained puzzled.

"I couldn't sleep at night or during the day," my dad says. "The lack of sleep caused drastic changes in my personality."

My dad is one of the calmest, most patient, most collected people I know. He worked exhausting night shifts as a jail guard to support our family and always made time for my siblings and me, never complaining when life got difficult. His quiet wisdom has helped me through many struggles in life. And yet, during this time, his personality changed. He was driving out to Winnipeg to pick up my mom one day (either he felt okay enough to be out that day or was forcing himself to function through the pain) and had to wait at an intersection for about fifteen minutes. He recalls that the wait made him so impatient, he had the urge to step out of the car and punch the cop who was directing traffic.

My dad wanted to hit a police officer. My. Dad. The idea of him getting even mildly annoyed for having to wait in traffic is unfathomable.

But chronic pain and exhaustion twist who we are, becoming such a powerful force that our emotions and state of mind are in turmoil. It's scary that our very personalities can be affected by constant pain and others may not understand or be patient with us through it (that police officer probably wouldn't have been very compassionate if my dad had actually hit him). Forget becoming a hero, sometimes we're just trying not to become a villain.

Thankfully, just as my dad reached for the door handle, he was struck by a moment of clarity and realized exactly how ridiculous his instinct was. He burst out laughing, able to comprehend that his emotions were warped from exhaustion, and stayed seated in the car until the cop motioned his vehicle forward.

"I understand how people in chronic pain can reach a breaking point and act irrationally," he says. "Thankfully, I did not have to spend any time in jail for assaulting a police officer to learn that."

But not everyone can pull it together like my dad did. If someone as patient as he is struggled with anger management, what about people who are more prone to rage in the first place? What about those who struggle with depression and anxiety even before chronic illness strikes? When we break down in front of those we love or snap at strangers on the street, we may not even understand the source of our emotions. Recognizing our own irrationality is a good first step to addressing this issue, and asking for grace is another.

I haven't personally wrestled with outbursts of anger like this. I struggle more with fear, withdrawing from the world when I don't know what else to do. When my body gets too tired, I just shut down. I feel like my personality has been replaced by a robot's, like I'm looking at myself from outside and don't recognize the person in my body. As a result, my behaviour toward others appears indifferent or cold. I may brush off a friend or make a sarcastic comment that is uncalled for.

While I'm not going to use pain as a scapegoat for my attitude, I can still consider its effect on my psyche. "Pain makes us make bad decisions," says Doctor House.[6] Pain is a huge motivator, and managing it can seem like an impossible task.

House's methods of management include yelling at people, avoiding relationships, becoming so obsessed with solving puzzles he doesn't care about the risks to his patients, making snarky comments, and abusing his position as a doctor by hoarding stashes of Vicodin and prescribing it to himself. I don't recommend any of these methods.

House's life is understandable, but it's sad, lonely, and chaotic. I don't want that kind of life. I'm willing to fight for peace. Some days that just means fighting to simply survive. And when the universal side effect of constant pain is exhaustion, "fighting" often means knowing when to stop pushing myself and taking time to rest.

4

GIVE IT ONE MILLION PERCENT

"Hollow cheeks and sunken eyes... to think that you're their greatest hero. Now the adoring public knows your true form. Try not to be ashamed."[1]

— ALL FOR ONE, *MY HERO ACADEMIA*

*L*ately, I've been afraid to go to bed. I've been having chronic vaginal pain that feels like a raging urinary tract infection, except doctors have run all the tests and don't know what's going on. The pain is more prevalent at night, and I'll huddle on the couch with a blanket, watching *The Office* for as long as my tired eyes will stay open.

If I go to bed, even though I'm exhausted, the pain seems worse because there's nothing to distract me from it while I try to fall asleep. The bed has become this horrifying symbol of my suffering, and peaceful sleep is difficult to come by.

At around 9:00 a.m., the pain starts to subside, and I

crawl into bed and sleep until the afternoon. I forced myself to go to dinner with friends one evening, where an acquaintance said how much she wished *she* could sleep in until noon. She doesn't understand she really does *not* want this.

I do not want to be bedridden. I would much rather be able to go about my daily life. My body is exhausted. My mind is exhausted. I've been wanting to get a haircut for three weeks, because it's been growing out of its pixie state into a mess that sticks up every which way, but I don't have the energy to leave the house. I've been skipping meetings, dates with friends, church, family dinners, and errands. I can't even stand up in the shower long enough to shave my legs—it's a quick soap up, rinse, and then get out, if I have the energy to shower at all.

SPOON THEORY

I said "I'm out of spoons" to my best friend when I told him I couldn't make it to church one night, and he dropped by that afternoon to give me a hug and a literal spoon. Now I have a nice reminder in the utensil drawer —one spoon unlike the others—that I have good people in my life who understand when I have to stay home. But not everyone is so understanding, because the constant drain is difficult to comprehend.

The Spoon Theory was created by Christine Miserandino, a lupus patient and founder of the website *But You Don't Look Sick*. She relates in a blog post how the analogy came up when she was having dinner with a friend, who asked her what it felt like to be sick all the time.

When mere words describing her pain didn't seem like enough, Christine gathered up a handful of spoons from nearby tables and handed them to her friend, telling her she now had hypothetical lupus.

The spoons represented how much energy Christine's friend had to work with for one imaginary day. Healthy people generally expect to have a never-ending supply of spoons, but sick people's spoons are limited. For every activity Christine's friend wanted to do for the day, she had to give up one of her twelve spoons. (Side note: I've seen memes that use spell slots in the roleplaying game Dungeons & Dragons to make this same analogy, and I love it. Never mind chronic illness warriors—we are chronic illness wizards!)

When Christine's friend started her day by getting ready for work, Christine took away one of the spoons and said, "No! You don't just get up. You have to crack open your eyes, and then realize you are late. You didn't sleep well the night before. You have to crawl out of bed, and then you have to make yourself something to eat before you can do anything else, because if you don't, you can't take your medicine, and if you don't take your medicine you might as well give up all your spoons for today and tomorrow too."[2]

When she hadn't even gotten to her hypothetical workplace yet and was down to six spoons, Christine's friend began to get a clearer picture of what living with lupus was like. Every chore, every activity, every outing took a spoon, and there weren't enough to do everything. She had to choose between eating dinner or running errands, because there weren't enough spoons for both. She could cook dinner, but then she'd be too tired to do the dishes. She could clean her apartment or do something fun, but she couldn't do both. By the end of the exercise, she was in tears of sympathy.

RATIONING YOUR SPOONS

The phrase "I'm tired" takes on a whole new meaning when you have a chronic condition.

Twenty-eight-year-old Emily has lupus too. She was diagnosed when she was nine. Lupus is a disease where your immune system attacks your own body, causing symptoms that can include fatigue, fever, joint pain, rashes, photosensitivity, chest pain, headaches, and confusion.

For Emily, the first symptoms were the "butterfly rash" on her face, something typical for lupus, and photosensitivity. Then the fatigue set in, along with a myriad of other painful issues. She was only able to attend school part-time and, even then, missed days regularly and ended up in the hospital almost every fall. After graduation, her situation improved because of a loving family who took care of her; she is currently able to manage her health because she doesn't have to work and can spend a lot of time doing what her body calls for—lots and lots of sleep.

"I'm not able to do the things I would like to, like taking my niece and nephew out," Emily said to me over a Facebook chat. "I would love to take them to the zoo, or museum, or something fun like that. But it takes so much energy, I can't do anything for at least a couple days, if not more."

Heading to the zoo for the afternoon may seem like a simple thing for most people, but for someone with a chronic condition, it can take an inordinate amount of mental and physical preparation for a short outing. Emily mentioned that just thinking about it is overwhelming. It's not just the outing itself that's exhausting; the planning, anticipation, and dread are tiring, too.

"I almost always have to plan a week ahead," Emily says. "I can't be spontaneous. It's like I need to pump myself up to go out or do any sort of activity. And I need to space things out; for instance, I volunteer at the humane society once a week. That's all I can do that day, even though it's just in the evening for two hours. I also need days in the week where I do nothing, just to recoup from whatever I've done the day before."

I'm not always good at planning out my week. Things seem to pile up, whether they're events, meetings, or outings to see friends I haven't visited in forever. Frequently, I'll get burnt out in the middle of the week and have to cancel whatever plans I had for the weekend. Even after more than twenty years of illness, I'm still not great at planning rest time, though I've been trying to get better at it. It's tricky, because some days I'll have energy and feel okay. On *those* days, I'll plan the other events, because *I feel fine! Of course I can manage!* And then I end up exhausting myself. It's important to factor rest days into my calendar—and lots of them.

JUST GIVE IT ONE MILLION PERCENT

In *My Hero Academia*, protagonist Midorya shouts, "One million percent!" before hitting an enemy, meaning he's giving the punch his all. He's trying to push past his limits to defeat a foe more powerful than he is. The math doesn't work, of course, since one hundred percent is all anyone can give.

With its mantra—"Go beyond! Plus Ultra!"—the show toys with the trope of finding extra strength within yourself. If you're losing a fight and finding yourself at the end of your powers, just try harder! There's a whole genre of this kind of anime, called *shonen*, from where the themes of "believe in yourself/friendship" and "find a hidden well of strength" originate. This idea is prevalent in a lot of American fiction, too, where the hero searches inside themself for the answer and gets an emotional jump-start at a crucial moment. It's a message I laugh at because there is no extra well of strength in me to find. Once I'm out, I'm out. No more spoons. If I could will myself to have more energy, I wouldn't; I'd will myself to be completely healed instead.

However, *My Hero Academia* redeems itself with its characterization of All Might, the world's Number One Hero and Symbol of Peace. He's not just the best superhero in the world, he's the superhero whose very presence has brought villains to their knees and who has ushered the world into veritable peace. All Might is also cripplingly sick; his respiratory system was severely damaged in a previous battle and, at the beginning of the show, he can only manage to keep his hero form for three hours a day. The tall, muscular image that the public knows is reduced to a scrawny, bleary-eyed guy for the rest of the time. The time he can spend in his hero state decreases as the show goes on and All Might stretches himself too thin.

At first, he acknowledges his progressing weakness and his desire to train Midorya as a successor by taking a teaching position at U.A. High, Midorya's school. But in the episode "Yeah, Just Do Your Best, Iida!" he can't help himself from stopping crime on the way to work. As a result, All Might's powers are all but depleted when he gets to class, and another teacher has to take over for him while he rests.

Maybe this wouldn't have been such a big deal if villains hadn't chosen that day to attack U.A. High.

All Might arrives to the fight a couple episodes later, with only a few minutes of his hero form left to attempt rescuing his students, several of whom are injured. He kicks himself for using up his powers earlier that day.

"I can't believe all this went down while I was resting," he says to himself.[3]

All Might pushes himself in the fight to save the students; he "goes beyond" and is able to beat back the enemy with the help of Midorya and friends. But he pays a price. Thereafter, the time he can spend fighting in his superhero form is reduced to fifty minutes.

All Might stopping to help people on his morning commute to work could be considered noble, and, in a way, it is. However, there were other heroes available who could have done what he did. He didn't need to deplete his powers before getting to his job, which severely hindered his ability to teach, something he had committed to. He prioritized his own image as a hero over training the next generation of heroes. I prioritize my own image over self-care sometimes too. I may not stop to solve crime like All Might, but I overextend myself, which leads to consequences later on.

LEARNING TO SAY NO

It's hard to let go of the self-reliant, helpful image I have of myself. In the past, I've said yes every time someone asked me to do something—whether it was volunteering at kids' camp, writing a press release, designing a poster, or editing a friend's novel, I was your woman. I've since learned that I can't do everything. I can't even do all the fun stuff I want to; this season, I had to choose between two regular outings—playing a Dungeons & Dragons campaign or singing in a choir… two things I love. I knew my body wouldn't be able to handle both.

I could push myself and try to do everything. And as I mentioned, sometimes I do. But that means borrowing spoons from tomorrow, and then the next day, and then the next. And pretty soon, I pay the toll for pushing myself beyond what I can manage and I crash.

Why do I push myself so hard? I'm not even fighting crime! It's not like the hope of the world rests on my scrawny shoulders. But I want to be doing the same things healthy people do. I want to be "normal." I want to be above normal—PLUS ULTRA!

In these early episodes of *My Hero Academia*, All Might instructs Midorya to pace himself and only use a small amount of his power because his prodigy could hurt himself by doing more. Midorya doesn't listen, and injures himself a lot in order to help others.

I'm not surprised that Midorya ignores his mentor's advice, because All Might doesn't practice what he preaches. All Might constantly pushes himself too far, sacrificing himself for the people around him. Midorya almost completely destroys his own hands by following his mentor's path.

If Midorya breaks his body, no matter how noble the cause, he won't be any good to anybody afterwards. He needs to take care of himself and recognize his limits.

The temptation to push myself is strong, whether it's because I feel cooped up, needy, guilty, or like a burden. Other times it's because I want to be there for the people I love; I want to be strong for them when they need me. But sometimes true strength is faithfully counting out your spoons and not going beyond your capacity for the day.

WITH GREAT ILLNESS COMES GREAT EXHAUSTIBILITY

People laugh when I say I'm tired if I get up any time after 10:00 in the morning. 9:00 a.m. is socially acceptable, though that's even pushing it for some. It's as if the fact that I've been awake until 4:00 a.m. with insomnia, restless legs, and whatever other pain issue I'm dealing with that day doesn't matter. *They* get up at 6:00 a.m. every day so the fact that I often sleep until noon is hilarious.

I've been working on feeling less guilty about my sleep patterns, because I can't control them. I'm very thankful that I work from home and have the freedom to sleep later. Not everyone has that advantage. I suspect sleep is an issue for most people with chronic pain or illness, though there is a specific chronic condition also related to exhaustion.

Chronic fatigue syndrome/myalgic encephalomyelitis (CFS/ME) is another one of those difficult-to-diagnose disorders because its cause is unknown, though there are studies that connect it to changes in immune function and cellular metabolism.[4] It's got a stigma to it, as some doctors don't believe it exists and many people misunderstand it with comments like, "Yeah, I'm tired too." The difference between regular exhaustion and CFS/ME is that sleep doesn't help the person with chronic fatigue. It can also be accompanied by joint pain, memory loss, and headaches. That's how Jennifer Brea, director of the documentary *Unrest*, describes her experience.

"When my neurologist diagnosed me, he said my symptoms were caused by a distant trauma, one I might not even remember," says Jennifer in the documentary. "So I walked home in spite of the pain in my legs, the burning in my brain. My body was screaming, but I ignored it because he told me 'this has no biological cause.'"[5]

She also relates the struggles she's had with feeling like her illness was swallowing her identity. People didn't understand what she was going through, and she wanted that to change.

Our identities are wrapped up in our activities, especially where we work. "So, what do you do for a living?" is the first question I ask to get to know someone. This knowledge helps me form a picture of who this person is, and I would feel lost if I wasn't able to begin with that icebreaker. Without it, it would feel like there's no base to the person I'm talking to. He's just hanging there by strings—not a "real boy" until I have a job title to associate with his name.

"What do you do for fun?" is another question I like to ask. I'm very lucky that I can do most of the things I love despite my illness. Writing, reading, gaming, and drawing are all possible activities for me, at least some of the time. However, it's when the illnesses pile on and I'm spending day after day on the couch, unable to even work on a computer, that I realize if I continue to define myself by what I can do, my identity comes up empty half the time.

I'm not just what I do. I'm not a collection of potential actions bundled up into a sack of bones and skin. Being a whole person means something more than that.

But if my identity isn't an editor, writer, volunteer, artist… what is it? Who am I when I'm too exhausted, too in pain to even get a haircut when I need one as badly as Chewbacca? The danger is that my identity and illness become tangled up, so I only think of myself as sick, tired, and worthless.

Mitch, an acquaintance in his forties, struggles with this question of identity much more than I do. A few years ago, he had complications during a spinal surgery, which included a stroke, and his left side was paralyzed. He informed me that our world is not designed for one-handed people.

"I can't do basic things in life," Mitch says. "Opening jars, opening a door... I haven't seen my basement in two years. Zippers are especially difficult. I've only recently been able to use the bathroom independently. Nothing quite like having two people join you in the bathroom each and every time you go."

Mitch says his confidence and self-esteem have taken a hit. He notices people literally talking over his head now, the outside world makes him nervous, and people doting over him without asking to help first frustrates him. Days at home mostly involve binge-watching TV shows he doesn't even like, because he's gone through so many of them.

Though being back at work part-time has helped his boredom and frustration, he still has to face a lot of failure. "In my recovery, I need to constantly try my limits, and my failures outweigh my successes. It's a hard pill to swallow to constantly try stuff out, mainly to fail," he says.

If I continue to define people by what they can do, that would mean categorizing Mitch as mainly a failure. But I can't do that, because I admire him for pushing forward through his condition. Even though it sucks, even though he may be depressed and frustrated most of the time, he's valuable. The world is a better place with him in it, even if all he's doing is binge-watching *The Brady Bunch.*

We focus so much on rating people according to their skills, talents, wealth, education, and social status that we forget they aren't items on a scale to be weighed for their worth. We forget that every person is unique and irreplaceable. We're not valuable because of what we do, we're valuable because of who we are. We're valuable because of our impossible-to-describe souls. We're valuable because we love and are loved.

FORGIVING YOURSELF

All Might loses everything familiar to him when he finally loses all his powers. No more hero form. He now has to learn to live in his powerless, scrawny body forever. It's quite an adjustment, especially when he's used to helping others and is unfamiliar with standing on the sidelines, or, heaven forbid, letting others help him.

All Might still has a lot to offer—to Midorya, his other

students, and the world. His experience makes him a valuable resource if he's willing to be patient and learn how to teach properly. But his life will not look the same. He has to learn to step back from the fight, to let others step up, to acknowledge his own weaknesses and make time for rest.

The world is going to change because of All Might's absence as a superhero. He was the Symbol of Peace and brought order to society. That peace will be threatened as villains realize he's gone and step in to cause chaos. Other superheroes will struggle to fill All Might's shoes and face pressure to accomplish the same things he did.

That future is probably playing through All Might's mind as he realizes his power has been depleted. He turns to the video camera that is broadcasting him live, points at the lens, and says, "Next, it's your turn."[6] While the message is meant for Midorya, the one who has inherited All Might's power, it can also be applied to all the young heroes. They need to step up. The burden is now theirs. All Might is all out of spoons.

There's no easy way to get through this transition, to give up the things you want to do but don't have the energy for, to say no, to invite others to take your place. Releasing the way you want life to be and accepting the way it is comes with frustration, anger, sadness, guilt, and a host of other emotions. The longing to do things I cannot do is strong. It's *plus ultra* strong.

It's frustrating when people expect me to manage things I cannot. It's worse when I expect those things of myself and am angry when I fail. I'm discovering it's easier when I offer grace to those people, and when I offer grace to myself. It's okay if I fail. It's okay if I can't do things other people can. It's okay if I'm weak and I let others be strong.

I feel like I should, somehow, be able to give one million percent, and I feel guilty that I can't. So I remind myself that my one hundred percent is good enough.

When errands go undone, when chores go unfinished, I tell myself it's all right. When I cancel plans with friends, when I take a three-hour nap, I forgive myself. When I'm depressed, when I'm exhausted, I give myself a little grace. I figure if I keep doing so, I'll eventually accept it. I can be unhappy about the number of spoons in my hand, but that doesn't mean I have to be angry at myself because I can't hold more. Like All Might, I'm learning to give up my image of strength for a reality that fits my body. I'm giving up the *plus ultra* life for a more peaceful existence.

5

FRIENDSHIP AND FIRE EMBLEM

"I hate being a burden on everyone."[1]

— RHYS, *FIRE EMBLEM: PATH OF RADIANCE*

I've always liked doing things for myself, without help from anyone. If I can't find what I'm looking for while I'm shopping, I'll spend a half-hour searching rather than ask a clerk for assistance. If I am lost, I will wander around aimlessly rather than ask for directions.

Being unable to figure things out for myself feels like failing. Relying on someone else feels like weakness. In his 1841 essay "Self-Reliance," Ralph Waldo Emerson writes, "Trust thyself: Every heart vibrates to that iron string." These words seem inspirational. Yes—iron! Iron is strong. I am strong and self-sufficient. *Rawr.*

The problem with chronic illness is that I cannot manage life by myself. Despite my desire to be self-sufficient, it's not always possible for someone who is ill.

Really, no one can do life on their own, even without the added burden of chronic illness. We are built to be inter-dependent.

SHARING THE BURDEN

I couldn't work much during university. I needed the financial support of my parents and from government student loans to attend. Years afterwards, I still needed my parents' help, and the generosity of others, to afford housing.

I relied on roommates and an understanding landlord to pay rent. After that, I lived in my friends' basement for several years, and because they are amazing people they charged me little rent. My life would have been pretty miserable if I hadn't let others assist in this way.

Though this dependency improved my quality of life, relying on others for financing still brings on feelings of guilt and shame. I feel like society expects me to be able to provide for myself, and I'm failing by not doing so.

Financial support isn't the only help I need. I often can't get to places I need to go or complete tasks that need doing, such as shopping for groceries, cooking meals, running errands, going to a doctor's appointment, moving to a new place, or changing a flat tire. I need physical support from friends and family to accomplish these things. Sometimes I just don't have the energy or physical strength to do them. I feel guilty when I ask someone else to run an errand for me because I'm too exhausted to leave the house.

In addition, I often rely on moral support from friends and family for the sake of my emotional health. I *could* go alone to doctor's appointments and emergency rooms, struggling through emotional issues by myself, but I'd be much less healthy for it. I especially find visits to the ER traumatizing and am grateful I've always had someone with me. Yet, I feel like "strength" is so often equated with going it on your own, like I am weak for relying on others in this way.

I've also benefited from spiritual support, which has been a key component in helping me cope with illness and life in general. Spirituality, which can include religion or not (in my case, it does), is about finding hope and meaning in life. Sometimes that hope sinks when I try to keep it afloat by myself, and others have to push it to the surface for me, whether by words of encouragement, reflective listening, or quiet company.

This financial, physical, moral, and spiritual support has been key to finding moments of peace through the storm of chronic illness—but for years, I struggled with asking for this help. I'd ask when I couldn't think of anything else to do, but I would feel guilty for doing so. And I often would refrain from asking for moral support at all, because that was the type of help that made me feel the weakest. As a result, I was physically taken care of, but there came a point in my life when I was so emotionally burdened I could hardly function.

LETTING GO OF PRIDE

I experienced a dark time in my life during my early twenties after I had moved away from my parents', but it was made manageable when I started attending a small group at my church. This was a group of people who seemed surprisingly comfortable sharing their burdens with each other. At first, I simply sat at these events, alone in my suffering, quiet, watching and listening to how they interacted with each other. We met in a family's living room, and the casualness, the fact that these people all seemed like friends and not just acquaintances who were there only to study the Bible, attracted me.

Every time someone brought up a topic they were struggling with, they were met with love, acceptance, and prayer. These three things were not foreign to me. Growing up as a church kid, I'd attended Bible studies, services, and youth groups that featured similar times of sharing and prayer. But I didn't feel safe in these circles. I was never one of the kids who spoke up and admitted I was going through something difficult. I kept my mouth shut, keeping my problems to myself, aware that these people were obligated to care for that half-hour, but after that, we weren't friends. They wouldn't follow up with me to see if I was okay—at least, I didn't believe they would. How was I, an introvert who wouldn't even open up to my mom about my issues when she asked, supposed to share my deepest emotional struggles with these people?

The other reason I didn't share was that I was too proud. I tried to look like a humble kid on the outside. But inside, I was too selfish to admit that I struggled to face my problems alone, that I was sick, that I was emotional, that I needed someone to share the burden with.

I don't know what changed with this new group. Maybe it was that they were involved in each other's lives *outside* of the weekly meetings, checking in with each other, going out to movies together, enjoying each other's company. They actually cared about each other, and they cared about me. Maybe it was that I'd finally hit rock bottom and I realized I'd rather have the help than my pride. Maybe it was a combination of the two.

"I'm missing too much work because I keep getting sick," I told the group one day. Though that may seem like a small personal detail, it was big for me to share *anything*. They met that acknowledgement with care and understanding, and I later admitted I was struggling with depression. I didn't feel an automatic rush of relief at sharing my feelings; in fact, I felt tense and strange, because I was so used to holding them in (and there was no taking it back once I said it). But eventually, I felt like my burden wasn't as heavy as it used to be. It wasn't lifted, but it was shared.

ASKING FOR HELP

In the video game *Fire Emblem: Path of Radiance*, Rhys is chronically ill. The game doesn't specify what his illness is, but he refers to frequently being in bed due to fever and shaking. Rhys is the healer of the party. His job is to use his magic staff to heal the cuts and bruises of his companions while they are in battle so they can continue fighting. It's ironic because Rhys can't use it to heal himself. Magic can't cure him.

In one scene, another character, Titania, asks Rhys if he'd be happier at home with his parents instead of travelling with their mercenary group. "Oh, I don't know," Rhys replies. "That life wasn't easy. I have a small, frail body, and there were few jobs for me in our village. My parents were always worried about me. I was sick all the time, and constantly getting bumps and scrapes.… They only agreed to let me follow you because you were a strong mercenary group! They figured I would be safe."

Rhys has found a place to belong with this group, a place where he is loved and accepted for who he is, illness and all, though it takes him some time to realize that. He struggles with feeling like a burden because of his illness. He doesn't want to hold anyone back or cause trouble when they have missions to carry out. When one of his other teammates, Rolf, notices that Rhys is looking pale, Rhys denies he is ill. Rolf calls him out on the lie, noting his hands are cold as ice.

> **Rhys:** …Sorry, Rolf. But I'm well enough to move around a battlefield, so I'll be all right.
> **Rolf:** You're talking about a battlefield, Rhys! Not some fort! Don't pretend to be fine if you're not! You'll end up dead if you keep doing stuff like that!
> **Rhys:** Rolf… I… I'm sorry…
> **Rolf:** Hmph!
> **Rhys**: I'm really sorry, Rolf. I wish… *Cough!* I wish I wasn't so frail. It would be nice to be strong.
> **Rolf:** Well, I wish your staff could heal sicknesses and not just big gaping axe wounds!
> **Rhys:** So do I… *Sigh* I wish I had a better plan than just waiting for it to pass.
> **Rolf:** Well, I'll ask Ike to let us fight together. At least then I can keep an eye on you.
> **Rhys:** Thanks, Rolf.

Though Rhys is trying not to be a burden by covering up his illness, Rolf is having none of it. Like so many people in my life who are willing to help me, Rolf is willing to help Rhys bear his burden. He cares about Rhys and doesn't see him as holding them back; Rolf considers Rhys an enhancement to his life and their group, not a detriment. As Rolf says in another conversation with Rhys, the mage "can't help being barfy all the time."

Asking for and accepting help is not weakness. When people tell me that I'm not a burden on them, I trust that they mean it. This doesn't mean they aren't going out of their way to help or that being there for me is always easy; it means that they are willing to do it. This also doesn't mean I'm all take and no give.

I don't want others to compare their suffering to mine and conclude mine is "worse." I don't want them to assume they can't come to me with their problems. I don't want friends to avoid mentioning they're having a difficult time at work or that they're sick with the flu. Everyone has problems and pain. Everyone needs support, and I can be there for others in the capacity that I am able.

Rhys wants to have purpose, and his staff allows him to contribute, to heal his party members when they need it. I have purpose too—everyone has gifts, talents, and abilities. If people treated me only as sick, those gifts die.

FRIENDS VS. CARETAKERS

If *all* I'm doing is moaning to my friends about my problems and fostering relationships where they don't feel comfortable bringing up anything about their own personal lives, but are only listening to mine, that's not a friendship; that's a psychologist and a patient.

While learning to let others take care of you is part of having a chronic condition, you can also swing too far to the other side of the pendulum and start using your illness as a crutch in your relationships. It's easy to use a chronic condition as an excuse to be selfish and tell yourself you're not *really* being selfish because you deserve to complain and to be listened to; your illness is so much worse than your friends' paltry problems, after all.

The problem is, weighing life circumstances like this is unfair. Suffering is suffering, and it doesn't need a number to quantify it. I can feel sad about the things my friends can do that I can't, but I can also celebrate their experiences with them at the same time.

In *Fire Emblem: Path of Radiance,* Rhys has a conversation with Ulki, a winged character:

Rhys: Say, you can really fly with those wings, huh?! I saw you turn into a hawk before… it was amazing! I envy you!

Ulki: Mrrr?

Rhys: Oh, sorry.… That probably sounds weird. I've always been sickly. When I was little, I spent a lot of time in bed. So… I used to gaze out the window and see all the little birds flying around the sky.… It must be fantastic! Flying wherever you want, whenever you want?!

Ulki: Um… Fantastic. Yes. I suppose. I never thought of it.

Rhys: Oh, I don't blame you! After all, you've been flying since you were born… soaring through the skies like a puffy cloud!

Rhys envies Ulki's ability to fly, something he wishes he could do—though his desire is tied to his illness and not just about being able to float in the sky. It's the freedom Ulki has that Rhys really wants.

Rhys's words to Ulki don't hide his longing, but they also aren't bitter. He's not complaining to Ulki, but pointing Ulki toward something he's taken for granted and admiring his friend's ability.

This is the type of attitude I try to adopt with my own friends. Sometimes I do need to complain, just like they need to rant to me about the horrible day they've had, but I consider friendship a give-and-take with people who are willing to make sacrifices for each other.

Like Rhys, I often feel like I'm a burden. But I've found the best friends are those who are willing to carry me and let me return the favour as much as I'm able.

REDEFINING FRIENDSHIP

I don't expect everyone to step up. The truth is, I *am* a burden on some people, a burden they're unwilling to carry. Just as I get tired of being sick, the people who care about me can get tired of my illness, too. Being around, and close to, someone who's sick a lot doesn't just mean you're willing to help out when they need it. It can also involve emotional stress that not everyone is prepared to deal with.

Seeing someone you love in pain a lot of the time has got to be difficult. Friends have described feeling helpless when I'm in pain and wishing they could do something about it. Generally, the only thing they can do is be present and be patient when I'm unavailable.

If the sickness is something that comes on later in life after relationships have been forged, people may feel like they "haven't signed up for this" and drift away from their sick friends. Some friendships are tied to specific activities, like playing sports, attending a weekly event or group, hiking, etc. When that activity is no longer possible for the sick person, the friendship may fizzle.

Whatever the reason, friendships collapsing due to illness can be incredibly heartbreaking because both people may feel abandoned or misunderstood by the other.

I'm tempted to call those who drift away selfish. I can't control what's happening to my body, after all, and it doesn't seem fair that they should leave me when I need them most.

"With the exception of a few people, everyone disappeared," writes Leanne Skarratt in an article on her blog, *Soul Over Sickness.*[2] Leanne lives with chronic fatigue syndrome/myalgic encephalomyelitis, severe anxiety, and a chronic skin condition, and she relates how friends deserted her when her illnesses got worse at eighteen. At the time, she felt incredibly let down.

But looking back, Leanne doesn't blame those people. "It's not that my friends didn't care, or that they had forgotten about me," she writes. "It's that society has a pretty narrow bandwidth when it comes to illness; either you recover or die. I think the concept of chronic, enduring conditions is still slightly outside the realm of public consciousness."

Like Leanne says, feeling abandoned isn't easy. But being in the shoes of the healthy person in the friendship isn't easy either.

When Nina's best friend, Charlotte, developed a chronic illness that kept her home most of the time, Nina hadn't expected their friendship to deteriorate.

Even though they live close to each other, Nina doesn't see her much anymore because Charlotte feels too sick to have someone over, even for a movie or something low key.

"Before then, we used to hang out every week," Nina says. "It's been really hard on her, and it's been hard for me too because I miss my friend."

Choosing topics to talk about when they chat is tricky, because Charlotte "gets too overwhelmed or it hits too close to home with her own battles and then she's falling apart and we both feel hurt."

> "I've mostly settled for listening to her, sharing basic life updates for me, and trying to just be a source where she can talk about stuff that makes her laugh," Nina says. "I feel selfish for even struggling with this—it would be so much easier for me if she just admitted that she can't be that person for this season of life. But the fact that she wants to be, but then I get hurt in the process, is a really hard spot, and then I feel bad for pulling back from sharing when I know that isn't what she wants."

Nina finds it especially difficult sharing news about her relationship with her boyfriend, because she knows Charlotte wants a romantic partner as well, but doesn't have the energy to spare.

When friendships like this fall apart due to illness, it's difficult to blame either party. Sometimes, neither person is equipped to handle such a severe change in circumstances. However, in Nina and Charlotte's case, they ended up redefining their relationship to make it work.

Several months after Nina voiced the above frustrations, she told me:

"Now, we see each other maybe every couple of months. But we text almost every day and talk over the phone to stay in touch. I've had to learn to keep conversations short, and to always be checking in, like, 'Are you up for talking right now?' And giving her an out when I sense she's tired, like 'Hey, I'm gonna let you rest, but I'm so glad we could talk.'"

When they do hang out, it's usually for about an hour before Charlotte needs to rest.

"In the past, we used to do things like watching movies, going out, or even travelling together… Now, I do things like help her get her groceries, or just come to her house so we can sit and talk in her room."

By redefining what their friendship looks like, Nina and Charlotte are able to have a relationship. It just took some work and considering the other person's needs.

Sickness changes your circumstances—your plans for your life, your job, your ability to do things you used to. Sickness impacts who you are as a person—your mental health, your ability to empathize, your perspective of the world. Friends may or may not be able to deal with either of those changes. I've learned to let go of the ones who cannot manage it and value close friendships with people willing to stay in my corner.

6

A DEPRESSED WOLF

"I'm not fit to help anyone. Not my family. Not my friends. Nobody."[1]

— CLOUD STRIFE, *FINAL FANTASY VII:*
ADVENT CHILDREN

*W*olves are my glorious, furry friends. At least, the fictional kind are. My patronus would be a wolf (I don't care that you say it's a sparrow, Pottermore). Wolf Link and Ghost are my heroes. In my first Dungeons & Dragons game, I played a druid because my character could turn into a wolf. I like the idea of a growly, ferocious-looking creature that's actually on the side of "good."

However, when a wolf appears in Cloud Strife's life in the movie *Advent Children*, it's a sign of anything but good. The wolf is connected to Cloud's emotional state, representing his depression and guilt.

Cloud's tale spans a series of video games, a movie,

and several short stories. In *Final Fantasy VII*, the video game in which he first appears, he experiences several traumatic events. In addition to being experimented on and confusing his memories with someone else's, he hurts his friend Aerith and then almost kills her while under the villain Sephiroth's influence. Later, he fails to prevent Aerith from dying in the iconic scene where Sephiroth drives his sword through her chest. I would be shocked if Cloud *didn't* exhibit some signs of trauma.

Interestingly enough, Cloud was never portrayed as a "strong" hero to begin with. *Final Fantasy VII* reveals that he struggled with motion sickness and lacked the physical aptitude to be considered for SOLDIER, the elite fighters of Shinra. He was ashamed of his status as a mere infantryman and wrestled with the decision to visit his mother when a mission took him to his home village.

At the end of *Final Fantasy VII*, Cloud overcomes Sephiroth's influence and helps save the world from being destroyed by a giant meteor. After the dust settles, he helps Tifa, his childhood friend, start a bar in a new city called Edge and runs a delivery service. They even take in two kids and become something of a family. You'd think Cloud would be content now that he has his proper memories, is safe, and is surrounded by people he loves. And he is. For a while. Until all the memories come flooding back.

Without Sephiroth and the world in peril to hold his concentration, all the emotions and pain Cloud keeps bottled up come bubbling out at the worst possible time— when he's trying to adjust to a new life.

In "The Case of Tifa," a short story in the collection *On the Way to a Smile*, Tifa starts to notice some changes in

Cloud. He becomes withdrawn (more so than usual) and doesn't come home very often. She finds a receipt from a delivery of flowers Cloud made to Aerith's grave, and it worries her because she knows he feels guilty about Aerith's death. At the end of the story, Cloud leaves and doesn't return, which is where the movie *Advent Children* picks up and when the wolf starts appearing in scenes relating to Cloud's mental distress.

In the movie, Tifa discovers Cloud has been hiding something else from her: he has contracted Geostigma, a disease sweeping across the world. The illness is incurable and results in weakness and open sores that ooze black goo. It also causes hallucinations, seizures, and pain in some of its victims. The wolf shows up in one scene where Cloud collapses from pain due to this illness.

Instead of relying on his loved ones for support, Cloud isolates himself, falling deeper into depression. The lone wolf is an apt metaphor for his psyche. He wants to be strong, but is afraid to be weak. He wants a family, but is afraid he is unlovable. He wants to be at peace, but feels anguish from his mental and physical illnesses.

"He chooses loneliness and death at the start of the movie because he's tired of hurting and doesn't believe that anyone should care about him," Emily Palmieri writes in an *Extra Life* article. "Tifa and Marlene's frustration with him mirrors the frustration and helplessness felt by loved ones of the mentally ill. Despite the fantastical world that Cloud lives in, he faces some of the most devastating and common of human problems."[2]

Cloud's response to pain is incredibly human; it's also incredibly common for people with chronic illnesses. I feel sad when I am weak, when I can't do the things I want to do, when emotions threaten to smother me. When this happens, the angst can spiral into depression.

SADNESS AND DEPRESSION

Sadness is when I long to go out to dinner with my friends, but have to stay home because I had an attack of stomach cramps. Sadness is when I wish I could be working on my latest book, but have to take a nap because I'm exhausted. Sadness is when I'm just starting to have a couple good days after a month of IBS lows, but then my period hits, and I'm struck with cramps again. Sadness is falling asleep sobbing because I just want the pain to stop already.

In contrast, depression is numbness, hopelessness, emptiness. Depression is when I sit on the couch, unable to figure out what to do with my day because none of the things that normally bring me joy sound the least bit interesting. Writing is futile. Painting is boring. Reading books takes too much concentration. Not even video games can entice me. Everything that gives my life meaning becomes meaningless. I *want* to want to do things. My sudden lack of interest is confusing, but my brain is foggy and I can't figure out why I don't care anymore. To keep up appearances of normalcy, I go through the motions, even though I can't recall why the motions are worth going through.

Sometimes, I become more irritable, because people around me interrupt my numbness by asking me stupid questions, like what I want for dinner. They don't understand I'm busy being numb and don't care about trivial things like food. Sometimes, I become more emotional and burst into tears at my own lack of desire to do anything. Sometimes, I just want to sleep, but I can't because the numbness forms a barrier between me and my dreams.

"I am, generally, an upbeat and positive person," says Derek, a minister who lives with IBS, joint pain, and chronic fatigue. "When my illnesses flare up, I can become very depressed. The depression can be over a number of factors: Can I really do my job? Take care of my family? Will people still put up with me? I often doubt my ability to be a useful and helpful person when battling illness. Recently, I've been diagnosed with arthritis in my back, and this is just another brick in the wall, which leads to doubting my self-worth."

Illnesses can impact mental health and can make us feel like we have no control over our own lives. I feel helpless when I can't force my emotions and my body into a normal state. I want my body and mind to submit, but they don't listen.

LEARNED HELPLESSNESS

In the late '60s and early '70s, psychologists Martin Seligman and Steven Maier conducted inhumane experiments on dogs that led to a theory about depression.[3] During one experiment, they divided the dogs into three groups: those in Group One were strapped into harnesses and did *not* receive any electric shocks; those in Group Two were strapped into harnesses and *did* receive shocks, but could end the shocks by pressing a panel with their noses; and those in Group Three were strapped into harnesses and received shocks, but were given no way to avoid them.

After this experiment, the researchers conducted another test, where the same dogs were placed, one at a time, in a box with a floor that shocked them but they could jump over a barrier into a shock-free zone. The dogs in Groups One and Two were quick to figure out how to avoid the shocks, but most of the dogs in Group Three wouldn't even try, lying down and whimpering instead. Because of their previous experience, they believed they were helpless to do anything about their pain.

When similar experiments were conducted on humans (but using stressors like loud sounds instead of electrical shocks), the results were the same. People learned helplessness when they were unable to control what was happening to them. Seligman identified two types of helplessness:

1) *Universal helplessness*, in which the subject believes nothing can be done about their situation.

2) *Personal helplessness*, in which the subject believes others could find a solution or avoid the pain, but they are personally incapable of doing so.

Both types of helplessness can exacerbate depression, but people who feel universal helplessness may blame external sources for their pain, and people with personal helplessness may blame themselves.

Those with chronic illnesses can suffer from either or both types of helplessness. I've experienced both. Sometimes I feel like there's nothing that can be done about my illness. Other times, I wonder if there *could* be something done about it—if researchers and doctors just put their minds to it and did more tests and funded studies—but, personally, I am incapable of doing anything about it. I often feel like, no matter what treatments or medications I try, nothing will help because that's the experience I've had so far.

I feel like one of those dogs, lying down and whimpering as I'm administered shocks, except not only is the cage closed, it is locked and barred. And there's a Behemoth King guarding the outside in case I ever manage to escape. But, while I can't solve my problems by discovering a medical solution to my illness and healing it, there are some things I can do to find peace through the feelings of hopelessness.

Even when there's no cure in sight, small pockets of joy can be found in life, whether it's simply making the most of a pain-free day or seeking solace in the company of a friend. There's a difference between acceptance and surrender.

MY HISTORY WITH DEPRESSION

I had an inkling I had problems with depression during my teenage years, and my parents did too. When my mom suggested I see a doctor or consider medication for it, I was adamant. "No. Absolutely not," I told her, and I refused to even discuss it. At the time, I didn't understand why tears welled in my eyes at the thought of taking an antidepressant. That was something other people did, and it was fine if they did it, but it wasn't the way for me. I was stronger than that. I didn't need it. I also didn't need to talk to anyone about my emotions, or even admit they existed.

Those were the lies I believed, anyway.

I made it through high school and university clinging to my denial. My depression was not severe enough for anyone to notice or force me to do something about it (i.e., I never harmed myself and wasn't suicidal). But it definitely made things much harder than they needed to be. I could muster up a normal demeanour in public, but I spent a lot of time on walks by myself, struggling to wrestle my emotions into submission. "I shouldn't be feeling like this" was a common thought for me, and I berated myself for feeling sad, guilty, angry, and numb. I took a lot of my frustrations out on my mom, sometimes replying to her loving attempts at conversation in a monotone with the fewest words possible and other times snapping at her. (Sorry, Mom.)

Depression often has zero discernible cause for the feelings it manifests. Either that or it exaggerates emotions and, even after the catalyst ceases to exist, continues to stick with you.

An estimated one third of people who struggle with chronic illnesses also struggle with depression.[4] The mind and body are linked, and it's no surprise that severe illnesses bring on mental challenges as well, what with all those feelings of hopelessness and worthlessness that sickness can bring about.

There came a point where I had to face my depression: I was triggered by an intense, emotional event that unearthed many factors that had been simmering below the surface. Interestingly enough, it wasn't my illness that was that catalyst (though that contributed largely to my feelings of worthlessness). It was a guy.

I went on my very first date *well* into adulthood, as my introvertedness, illness, and whatever other random-ness kept me from doing so in the past. At that point, I was out of university, working and living on my own. (Sort of. I had roommates.) I made friends with this guy, and I was captivated, especially since he seemed to like me and all my gaming nerdiness. He asked me out, and I was elated. Of course, I said yes.

The date was awkward, since I'd never been on one and didn't know how to act, but I had fun. He was incredibly smart and funny, with a dark sarcasm that made me giggle. I liked him. I wanted more.

He never asked me out again.

But we were friends, so I still saw him a lot. He seemed to enjoy my company, and I liked his, so I kept waiting for him to ask me on a second date. When it didn't come, I started to question whether that had been a date in the first place. Had he actually asked me out? Had he even used the word *date*? Had I misinterpreted everything?

I started second-guessing everything I did around him, playing conversations we'd had over and over in my mind and rehearsing new ones. Should I just ask him if it had been a date? And if he said yes, should I ask him why he hadn't asked me out again? What didn't he like about me? Wasn't I good enough?

I was confused why he never mentioned it. I was self-conscious. I was angry with myself for being unable to get over it. I felt worthless. Plus, I was new to dating and came from a conservative Christian background, so I didn't understand that going on a date wasn't necessarily meaningful. It's trying something out, and if it doesn't work out, that's okay. But for me, at that time, it felt like the end of the world.

My unrequited feelings and struggles with worthlessness revealed some deep-seated emotional issues. I progressed down a spiral over a two-year period that brought me to the point where I was in so much anguish it was affecting my physical health, my appetite, and my sleep.

I realized I had to stop being friends with this guy, since I couldn't seem to get a handle on my emotions. I had never had to tell someone we couldn't be friends anymore, and to this day it is the hardest thing I have ever done (though, like a coward, I sent him a message instead of telling him in person). I value loyalty and friendship over most things, and telling someone I cared about that I just couldn't deal with it felt like an incredible failure on my part. What was wrong with me, that I couldn't get rid of these feelings?

During this time, I went through episodes of numbness and then periods of intense emotion. I remember crying as I stared out the window into our backyard while I washed dishes. I remember crying while I tried to fall asleep. I remember crying at the office and hiding my tears from co-workers. My IBS was awful too, because my body didn't have the strength to deal with it on top of everything else. I especially dealt with nausea during this time, my roiling stomach often holding back the veil of sleep, refusing to let me out of my misery, so I was a bleary-eyed mess in the mornings.

No one knew what I was going through except two of my best friends, and I don't remember exactly how much they knew (a lot of that time is foggy for me). They counselled me to see a professional, and I must have listened, because I distinctly remember sobbing in my doctor's office as she handed me a box of tissues and prescribed me an antidepressant.

The antidepressant helped, though my mental health's improvement was a vertical climb at a sloth's pace. I wasn't resistant to taking meds once the bottle was in my hand—because I felt like I had lost a battle and was resigned to my defeat.

However, eventually I became more open about my emotional struggles with people close to me, admitting I was struggling in the first place and letting myself be vulnerable. Contrary to my belief, people didn't shove me out of their lives for being "weak." They accepted me for being human. I developed deeper relationships with friends than I'd ever had in the past because I wasn't masquerading as an emotionless woman who had it all together. I learned who the valuable people were in my life and met some new friends who made a space for me and my depression. That space gave me time to heal.

DISCARDING GUILT, ACCEPTING LOVE

In *Advent Children*, Cloud retreats into isolation, but he is never really alone. Various scenes show him listening to his friends' messages on his phone and receiving divine assistance from Aerith. All of his friends show up to assist him in a battle against Sephiroth's minions and Bahamut, a ginormous dragon whose breath is an energy beam of destruction. At this point in the movie, Cloud is incredibly calm and appears to be at peace with himself; he's come to a point where he has realized he is stronger with his friends by his side.

He strikes Bahamut on his own, forcing the dragon to the ground, but the monster gets up again and heads straight for the skies.

Most of the scenes up to this point have featured characters who are lonely—Cloud on motorcycle chases with the villains, Tifa wondering where Cloud is and fighting on her own to protect her adopted daughter, deserted children being captured and enslaved. Isolating himself impacts not only Cloud, but those closest to him.

In this climactic reunion, however, Cloud's friends gather together. His buddy Barret literally gives him a boost so Cloud can follow Bahamut upward and strike once more. When Bahamut shoves him down, another friend appears to launch Cloud skyward. As the dragon travels to impossible heights, more friends appear to boost him up, and Cloud pierces through Bahamut's breath weapon. Aerith's spirit is the final hand that launches him one more time, and he is able deliver the final blow to the beast. Sure, the physics don't work, but it's emotional magic.

The wolf appears again at the end of the movie, as Aerith and Zack's spirits show up in a heart-warming moment. Then the animal disappears, symbolizing Cloud forgiving himself, letting go of his feelings of guilt and worthlessness.

Though depression may still hit him again later on, the burden of responsibility is gone. The shame is lifted. It's a crushing weight to bear by yourself, especially when your friends say that you don't need to carry it at all.

I still experience depression, but like Cloud, I no

longer associate it with guilt. I no longer feel like my emotions are my fault, like it's my responsibility to beat them into submission. I no longer feel like I'm letting people down because of something I have no power over.

In *Advent Children*, Tifa comments that Cloud found the strength to fight again. That strength did not come from some inner well of power, but from making peace with himself and allowing others to love him. Sometimes I find Cloud's smile and contented look on my own face when I do the same. When I stop blaming myself, the wolf fades away.

7

IN SICKNESS AND UNHEALTH

"This time tomorrow, the owls will start arriving from parents—they will not want a werewolf teaching their children, Harry."[1]

— REMUS LUPIN, *HARRY POTTER AND THE PRISONER OF AZKABAN* BY J. K. ROWLING

*R*emus Lupin is one of my favourite Harry Potter characters, and not just because he's part wolf. Along with being the only Defense Against the Dark Arts professor who's competent and genuinely cares about his students, Lupin demonstrates a self-consciousness I can relate to. Lupin is wise, kind, and thoughtful. Oh, and he turns into a vicious creature during the full moon. NBD.

J. K. Rowling[2] intended the character to represent the stigma surrounding blood disorders like HIV and AIDS. Lupin wears the only shabby clothes he can afford and doesn't have a steady job because of the prejudice over his condition.

He's a humble character, calmly leaving his job at Hogwarts at the end of Harry's third year because word spreads he's a werewolf. However, in *Harry Potter and the Half-Blood Prince* it becomes clear how little Lupin thinks of himself. He spends most of the book avoiding the witch he loves because he thinks she could do better than him. His humility isn't the healthy kind, but is steeped in low self-worth and the refusal to accept that anyone might love him the way he is.

Lupin was bitten as a child because his father, Lyall Lupin, publicly called werewolves soulless and evil in front of Fenrir Greyback, a savage werewolf. Greyback retaliated by turning Lyall's son into a werewolf, and Lyall had to confront his own prejudice:

> "[Lyall] had parroted what was the common view of werewolves in his community, but his son was what he had always been—loveable and clever—except for that terrible period at the full moon when he suffered an excruciating transformation and became a danger to everyone around him."[3]

Though his father's perspective about werewolves changed when he was personally invested in one, Lupin's opinion of himself is steeped in others' treatment of him. It's why, when he falls in love with Nymphadora Tonks, he refuses to believe she might love him back. When Tonks makes a remark about Sirius Black's good looks, Lupin responds with a bitter quip about him always getting women.

"You'd know perfectly well who I've fallen for, if you weren't too busy feeling sorry for yourself to notice," Tonks replies angrily.[4]

Even after Lupin realizes Tonks loves him back, he pushes her away because he thinks she deserves better.

AFRAID OF REJECTION

Lupin's attitude represents a real issue faced by people struggling with chronic illness; dating requires vulnerability, which can lead to rejection, which can damage self-esteem. Illness adds another complicated layer to romance because not everyone is prepared or willing to date someone who is sick all the time. I was less willing to test the waters because my self-esteem had already taken several hits from friends, family, doctors, and my own fear.

I badly wanted to date when I was in high school. No one asked me out, possibly because I was a bit of a nerd, possibly because I attended a Christian high school with about fifty students, and possibly because many of the guys I knew had adopted the *I Kissed Dating Goodbye* mentality (from a book that spread like wildfire through Christian circles in the early 2000s purporting that hearts should be "guarded," dating is dangerous, and you should wait for the "one"). I'm glad now I didn't date in high school, because I would have hidden my illness, and the effort of doing so would have stressed me out. But at the time, I watched other high schoolers pair off and, as Rowling would put it, "snog each other" in the locker room, and I felt jealous. I wished someone wanted me that way.

Later, as a young adult in university when my condition worsened, the idea of dating seemed impossible. How did one even find the time between school and being sick, much less the willingness to let a romantic interest know that if I disappeared to the bathroom for a half-hour during dinner, it was totally normal?

Wanting to date but choosing not to because your body is too exhausted is a perfectly legitimate response, but it's also draining. I wanted a partner. I wanted someone to share the burden, not to be my caretaker, but to live life with. I longed for physical touch—someone to hold me when I was in pain, to hug me when I didn't think I could take it anymore. And I wanted to be there for someone else too. I was capable of being a loving partner in return; my baggage just took the form of an invisible illness.

Even if I hadn't been dealing with so much fatigue, I may have been too scared to date in college. What if I was interested in a guy, but then kept cancelling on him because I wasn't feeling well enough? (Which, let's be honest, would happen. A lot.) How long would he keep believing me when I told him I was still interested? Would he agree to a fifth date after I'd cancelled the last three? Would he move on because dating me was so much work?

The few crushes that I did have over those years—friendships that developed mostly over email and online gaming—were met with rejection, which certainly didn't help my self-esteem. It also didn't help that I had already rejected myself.

As the years went by, I graduated from university and some of my symptoms became more manageable thanks to medication. But it seemed like all the guys I met who were mature enough to handle my illness were already married or dating. Of course, there's more to that story than just the "good ones being taken."

I was looking for someone very specific—someone who shared my religious faith, was mature, loving, open to *not* having children, and willing to understand (and sign up for) chronic illness. Plus, on top of all that, I wanted to be attracted to him. I wanted there to be a spark, not just check marks on a list. In the few short relationships I had during my early twenties, I compromised a lot out of a mix of hope and desperation. I rarely brought up my condition because I was afraid that it would drive them away—and also afraid that I might get too attached. Why trust someone with that intimate knowledge when they were just going to leave me?

Deep down, I didn't think I was worthy of romantic love. After the dust settled from a breakup, I would think, "I'm not worth it so there's no point in even trying," and I would give up looking for a while.

"Feeling like a medical specimen is decidedly unsexy, somehow the opposite of whatever we're taught is womanhood," writes Michele Lent Hirsch in her book *Invisible.*[5] Michele discusses her own feelings of inadequacy and relates having to stop herself from apologizing to her boyfriend for her pain.

"Why would you apologize for your body hurting?" he asked her, a completely logical question. But I understand her inclination to do so. I understand why the apology slipped out, why someone would feel like they needed to ask forgiveness for the inconvenience they were causing.

I tried to convince myself I was valuable, I was worth something, I had talents and abilities, plus a chill personality. Friends told me I was a catch and didn't understand why I was single for so long. I nodded along with them. Sure, I was "great." I deserved someone. Yet, secretly, I asked myself why someone would choose to be with me when they could be with someone healthy.

HEALTHY/ATHLETIC/LOVES TRAVEL

Online dating is a decent option for people with health issues. I could surf through waves of potential dates from the comfort of my computer chair. However, I couldn't handle the icky feelings when guys kept messaging me with openers like, "Ur hot," and, "Sex tonight?" I reached out a few times to potential guys but got no response; had a few so-so conversations; made one Facebook friend who was super nice but lived too far away; and went on zero actual dates. The lack of in-person dates was more a result of my own fears, uncertainty, and disillusionment than the format itself.

I remember pulling out my phone and thinking, "I'll give this another try. I've got this," and scrolling through the meat market of men that was this thing called Tinder (or Match, or eHarmony, or whatever site I was on). Left, right, left, right. I started to look more closely at what their interests were in a potential mate.

"Active."

Ugh.

"Loves adventure! Travel! The outdoors!"

Oh no.

"Athletic. Healthy."

I'm going to be single for the rest of my life.

Here I am: unhealthy, often inactive due to pain, definitely not athletic. Travelling makes me nervous because I never know when I'm going to be hit with an attack. I'm not big on camping or the outdoors because of... well, let's face it: the lack of spider-free bathrooms.

Reading these expectations over and over again, I felt out of commission. I didn't fit the criteria.

My insecurities and exhaustion led me to cancel my profiles after a mere month. I just didn't have enough energy to wade through all the data and try to discern whether a guy was legitimately interested in a relationship or not. A month definitely is not enough time to give online dating a real chance, but I was done with looking.

I greatly admire my single friends who persevere through multiple dating sites. Many of them have shared online dating stories with me that sound like they're straight out of a sitcom, including a ditty about one guy who required that his future wife be a good cook, homeschool their children, be submissive, healthy, active, loyal... the list went on (including a lengthy bit about making a dress look good on Sunday morning and preferring exercise to Netflix).

I'll take Netflix over a Sunday-morning dress any day, thank you very much.

I certainly wasn't interested in dating anyone with a list like this, and my self-esteem told me "healthy" was on everyone's list, explicitly stated or not.

I know there are decent people with appropriate expectations in the online-dating world, because friends have also shared positive stories with me. They've met spouses and gone on to have healthy relationships through online dating. It just wasn't the platform for me at a time when my insecurities shackled me from giving it a chance.

THE BLIND DATE

After I had come out of a year-long crush where I'd been rejected after admitting my feelings and a one-month relationship where I'd been dumped, I jokingly told my best friend, Kyle, that he could have control over my love life.

Apparently, he took me seriously, because a few weeks later, as we were setting up recording equipment for a podcast we co-hosted together, he told me he knew a guy I might like. He was willing to set us up if I was interested.

Nervousness swirled in the pit of my stomach. "No, thanks," I replied. Blind dates were nerve-wracking, and I was tired of looking for a partner anyway.

But apparently I wasn't *that* tired, because I was soon in a sort-of online relationship/friendship/it's-complicated-ship. It only lasted for a few months, after which I called things off because it was too stressful. And then I was done. Enough was enough. I was going to be single forever, and I was FINE with it. So fine.

It was fine.

Except Kyle suspected I really wasn't fine; I was lonely. He brought up the blind date prospect again. When I told him blind dates made me nervous, he suggested we go on a double date with him and his wife, whom I was also good friends with. We could go to a board game café, and it would be super chill.

I believe my words were, "Okay, fine."

Of course, Kyle wouldn't tell me anything about this guy, not even his name, before our date. He was trying to pique my curiosity so that I'd feel excited instead of nervous. Or at least excited *as well as* nervous. Sneaky, Kyle. Sneaky. It worked. Now that I'd said yes, I *was* curious. Kyle knew all my traits, quirks, passions, and flaws, and he understood the stress my illness put on me; I started to wonder what kind of guy he thought I would get along with. I even started bugging him to schedule the date so that I could put it in my calendar, though I still didn't have high hopes for it. That's what I told myself, anyway.

A week before the date, I attended a book study that a pastor friend invited me to. A couple of people were already there when I arrived, and I sat down on a couch next to a guy I vaguely recognized because we had attended some of the same events in the past. Jordan was a youth leader at my church and played in a Dungeons & Dragons game with some of the kids, so our conversation easily flowed; we discussed D&D character classes (I played a bard and he played a cleric) and what our favourite spells were.

I normally feel uncomfortable when I meet new people but was oddly at ease chatting with him. He reminded me of Oz from *Buffy the Vampire Slayer*—very chill. We talked non-stop until we were forced to shush because other people arrived and the meeting started.

As the night went on and I heard him contribute intelligently to the conversation, I started to feel attracted to this stranger. In fact, I remember that at one point the thought flitted unbidden through my mind of how nice it would feel to have this guy's arm around me. And my next thought was: *Where did* that *come from? I've just MET this guy!*

I chuckled to myself at the absurdity of what was obviously just a random emotion. I wasn't even sure if he was single. (Did I peek at his hands to see if he was wearing a wedding ring? You'll never know.) Plus, I shouldn't pursue anything anyway because I had promised to go on the blind date, and I didn't want to be distracted for it.

But what were the odds I would so easily jive with the guy Kyle had picked? That didn't happen very often. I was pretty sure Kyle knew Jordan, too. Maybe if the blind date didn't work out, I could ask Kyle to please set me up with him instead?

The night of the date rolled around, and I trudged through wintry night air, the kind where your breath turns to ice, to get to the board game lounge. My nerves increased with every snow-crunching step. I really didn't want to do this. Why was I doing this again?

As the rush of warm air greeted me when I opened the door, I scanned the room, which was filled with mostly empty tables and lined with shelves of board games. There was Kyle, standing beside a shelf with a game in his hand—Tsuro of the Seas, in case you were wondering—and chatting with none other than... Jordan. My hesitation melted like the ice crusting my eyelashes.

Jordan turned to look at me calmly (though I later learned he was nervous, too).

"We already know each other!" I blurted out instead of just saying hi. Smooth.

I was still nervous but cautiously intrigued as the date went on. After we played a few rounds of Tsuro, Kyle and Marilyn had to leave because their babysitter was only available until 9:00 p.m. That's the weak excuse they gave, anyway.

Jordan and I stayed, playing Seven Wonders and chatting until late evening. We discussed everything from our families to our favourite shows, and had he seen *Thor: Ragnarok* yet? Because it was magnificent, and he really should (hint: I'd be totally willing to see it again, it was *that* good). He casually mentioned he listened to the podcast I co-hosted. I remember having a sore neck by the end of the evening from leaning forward in my seat, because a large group of noisy gamers had come in and made it hard for us to hear each other.

At the end of the date, we walked together part of the way to my car and then separated. Despite my comfort in his presence, I wasn't head-over-heels, love-at-first-sight attracted, but I was interested in going on another date. Except he had been so difficult to read; I had no idea if he was into me or not. Also, I hadn't brought up my illness at all. And it was important he know about it. When should I tell him? Best to wait and see if he was interested first. If he was… the second date seemed too soon. The third date… well, if we're having a good time, it'd be a shame to spoil it with serious conversation. Fourth… is that too late? What if I get sick and have to hide it because I haven't told him yet? Fifth… I should definitely tell him by then, right?

Wait.

He had mentioned listening to the podcast… a podcast where we had done an episode about sickness and disability in fiction and I had talked about my illness.

He already knew.

He had known going in.

I mean, he didn't know the gory details, but he had an inkling. That was… kinda cool. Also, totally unfair! He knew all these personal details about me from listening to the podcast, and I knew next to nothing about him!

I messaged him to rectify the situation, and we chatted online almost non-stop for the next week, after which he asked me out to dinner, and our dating relationship began.

DATING WITH AN ILLNESS

In her book *Aches, Pains, and Love*, Kira Lynne writes that she was diagnosed with vulvodynia at twenty, and a specialist told her that she "would never be able to have a successful marriage or intimate relationship."[6] Imagine hearing that from a doctor—someone most of us would consider an authority on the matter; I would have believed it, and so did Kira.

Vulvodynia is pain in the vagina, which can include burning, soreness, stinging, itching, and painful intercourse, with no identifiable cause. Like IBS, doctors don't know why it happens, and women just have to live with it.

In her book, Kira describes being in denial about her condition before diagnosis—she persisted in riding horses, wearing tight pants, and having sex despite pain that lasted for days or weeks after these activities. Even after seeing the specialist, she hoped it would get better, but it only got worse in her thirties as she was hit with several more conditions and more pain.

She writes, "I felt that I had been robbed not only of a pain-free life, a life where I could be physically active and work full-time (or at all), but also of a life with a boyfriend, partner, husband, whatever you want to call him. I had been robbed of romance and love and affection. I felt like so much had been taken away from me."[7]

But Kira, after longing for a successful relationship through her twenties and most of her thirties, came to the realization that she didn't have to hold on to the misguided belief her doctor had forced upon her. The search for a partner may be tougher for her than for others, but it wasn't impossible.

THOUGH A DOCTOR never said I couldn't date, I carried similar feelings of worthlessness with me into my relationship with Jordan. Even though he knew I had physical problems, knowing was different than experiencing. I dreaded the day he would witness my weakness. And, of course, that day came early on.

On our third date, I had come to his condo to eat dinner and watch the TV show *RWBY* with him. But sitting on the couch after dinner, I was suddenly overcome with nausea. This happens to me sometimes— another anomaly of my deficient body.

The idea of barfing in front of Jordan, even the idea of just feeling sick around him, was completely embarrassing. I tried to stay upright without saying anything. I wondered what excuse I could make up for bolting out of his condo early, but then realized I probably couldn't drive home safely. I completely missed Ruby's fiery encounter with Weiss at Beacon Academy because all I could think about was the swirling motion of my woozy tummy.

But if I was to continue dating him, he was going to see stuff like this eventually. Might as well be honest and hope he takes it okay. So I admitted I was sick and needed to lie down. He was so sweet about it, helping me to his bed, grabbing me a pail in case I needed to puke, and rubbing my back as I miserably lay on his mattress until the nausea eased up. Best date ever.

There was no awkwardness, though; there was no look of disgust on his face. And that was the perfect response: kind, loving, accepting.

After that date, instead of relief, anxiety started to set in. I started to panic because I was beginning to fall for this guy. And what if, after the hundredth time I was sick, he got tired of it and realized he wasn't willing to deal with it after all? What if his love of travelling was greater than his feelings for me, and he decided he didn't want to be tied down by an unhealthy person? What if I wasn't going to have the energy to have as much sex as he wanted? If I continued to get close to him and he changed his mind later, I would have to deal with the emotional fallout of rejection. I was tempted to just run away from the relationship before that happened.

I was completely overcome by panic as I walked to his car before another date. The scene is forever imprinted on my mind—the crunching of my boots on the snow; the dark, wintry sky; watching my breath mist the air as the cold crept beneath my jacket; the smell of exhaust as I climbed in the car. But mostly, I remember the barrage of emotions and several overwhelming thoughts telling me to turn around and go back into the warm house: *What do you think you're doing? It's not worth it.* I had to force my legs to keep moving and mostly did so because the embarrassment of cancelling a date in person was too much. If I could just get through the evening, I could always end things later.

But I didn't end things, because, though I was scared, his steadfastness and compassion made me feel safe. He didn't push me to go somewhere when I wasn't feeling well or to do anything I didn't want to do. He was fine with staying in and watching Netflix or playing video games together—in fact, that was his preference. He was nonplussed when I sheepishly asked him if he would be willing to switch to unscented laundry detergent and deodorant because I had allergies and my eyes were itchy and watery after cuddling with him. Talk about an awkward thing to ask! It sounds like a simple request, but it's really weird asking someone to change their routine for you. Of course, he was perfectly happy to do so.

I kept wondering whenever I brought up a new health issue—whether it was allergies, iron deficiency, frequent bladder infections, or some future problem I was currently unaware of—if it would be the last straw.

But it never was.

He didn't get scared away. He didn't leave my side. He wanted me. Just me. And he was so sure about it, he asked me to marry him. (Spoiler alert: I said yes, and we had a delightfully nerdy wedding that included a Scripture reading in Elvish, board games, chocolate frogs, and centrepieces made with D&D dice.)

IN SICKNESS AND UNHEALTH

In *Harry Potter and the Half-Blood Prince*, the werewolf Greyback bites Bill, Ron's brother, during a battle.

Though it isn't a full moon during the fight, Bill is physically scarred and forever changed. As Bill lies in a hospital bed with his family surrounding him, Mrs. Weasley laments that he had always been so handsome, and now his face is scarred. "And he was g-going to be married!" she sobs. Fleur, Bill's fiancé, turns to her and demands what she means. "You thought I would not weesh to marry him? Or per'aps, you 'oped?" she says.[8]

Part Veela, Fleur is known for her beauty and overwhelming personality, and Mrs. Weasley wrongly assumes that Bill's appearance—and whatever other side effects the werewolf bite inflicted—matters to her. But Fleur is more mature than Mrs. Weasley gives her credit for; she genuinely loves Bill, all of who he is and who he will become.

Lupin and Tonks witness this exchange, finally facing the main issue standing between them—not Lupin's illness, but his unwillingness to let someone else accept him:

> "You see!" said a strained voice. Tonks was glaring at Lupin. "She still wants to marry him, even though he's been bitten! She doesn't care!"
>
> "It's different," said Lupin, barely moving his lips and looking suddenly tense. "Bill will not be a full werewolf. The cases are completely—"
>
> "But I don't care either, I don't care!" said Tonks, seizing the front of Lupin's robes and shaking them. "I've told you a million times…"
>
> "And I've told *you* a million times," said Lupin, refusing to meet her eyes, staring at the floor, "that I am too old for you, too poor… too dangerous…"

> "I've said all along you're taking a ridiculous line on this, Remus," said Mrs. Weasley over Fleur's shoulder as she patted her on the back.
>
> "I am not being ridiculous," said Lupin steadily. "Tonks deserves somebody young and whole."
>
> "But she wants you," said Mr. Weasley, with a small smile. "And after all, Remus, young and whole men do not necessarily remain so."[9]

I jokingly refer to the line Jordan and I said in our marriage vows as "in sickness and unhealth" because that's a more apt description of what he agreed to. People should think deeply about what that means when they say it, because, like Mr. Weasley says, healthy people do not necessarily remain that way. Our imperfect bodies fail us all the time, and real love means acknowledging that reality and devoting yourself to the other person. I know it's not easy for Jordan to see someone he loves in pain regularly. But his wedding vows weren't just mere words —he meant them.

No relationship or marriage is perfect, and ours is no exception, but I've experienced a lot of joy despite my suffering because of a loving partner who accepts me as I am.

I am painfully aware of the loneliness singleness can inflict when you desperately want to be married. The difficulties of being single *and* sick only add to that frustration. My joy from our relationship does *not* mean that my years spent as a single person were just stepping stones to get to this point or that single people with chronic conditions cannot find fulfillment. I may have struggled with loneliness when I was single, but I was still a whole person working toward making peace with life and my illness.

Jordan and I were not two sides of the same coin that were only complete when we found each other; we were (and are) two separate people who have communities that support us—and we would have been okay remaining single. We do think we're better together; I like being someone's priority, and several emotions I struggled with before, like loneliness, are easier to manage. Loving somebody who loves you back feels wonderful. Plus, I have a free foot-warmer in my bed every night.

However, I completely understand people who are simply too exhausted, or in too much pain, to desire a relationship. I know several people who have said they just can't muster up the energy to date. "I'd rather stick with celibacy than have to tell someone I've brought home that I'm terribly sorry, but I have to go spend the night in the bathroom, or that my pain level is suddenly such that I can't bear to be touched," says Kate, who suffers from nerve damage, IBS, arthritis, and anxiety. "I've decided there isn't a single person who would meet all my nitpicky, emotionally and physically damaged standards, and I absolutely refuse to 'just settle.'"

Others want badly to find a partner, but just can't imagine how it would work or who could accept them. "I feel guilty about inviting someone into this chronic issue," says Lindsay, who wrestles with nerve pain. "I didn't choose this, but they do.... Most of the time I feel hopeless when it comes to romantic relationships. However, I have close friends who have reminded me even this week that they are willing to walk with me and share the burden. So maybe?"

Healthy friends and communities can help bear the weight of singleness. Of course, most communities (in my experience, especially churches) focus on only a few factors when bringing people together—age, gender, or marital status—using any social mixers for singles as an excuse to set them up. I often find myself screaming into the void that there should be space for singles who are suffering, not just attempts to marry them off. Forging platonic relationships and learning ways to manage singleness (and illness) are more than needed.

It's difficult being sick, whatever your relationship status. It's a challenge when you badly want a partner but feel like you're unlovable. I understand why Lupin waited so long to let Tonks in. I understand why people lose hope that they will ever be able to find someone like Tonks (or Jordan) with whom to live their lives. And I can't guarantee that they will. I can't guarantee that if you just keep looking, you will find a partner. All I can guarantee is that there is hope and that sick people are worthy of every kind of love. My body might be broken, but it is not worthless and it is not unlovable.

To all the sick people out there, remember this—you are lovable. You are valuable. You are worth it. Your body, your love, and your existence matter.

8

THE QUESTION OF CHILDREN

"I can't ever give you children."[1]

— AMY POND, *DOCTOR WHO*

W hen we were initially getting to know each other, Jordan and I would play the "random question game" over text, where we'd take turns asking each other anything from "What's your favourite colour?" to "What's your biggest fear?" One day, he messaged: "You seem to be friends with lots of people with kids. Do you want some of your own some day?"

I waited for my heart to start up again before responding. I'd been dreading this question and struggled to bring it up myself because I knew if our answers differed, our relationship could come crashing down.

My answer was no. Though the way I phrased it was "I don't think I necessarily do"—because if my answer is wordy, it makes it less official, right? Maybe he wouldn't think I was a child-hating monster this way.

I had contemplated my answer to this question well before meeting him, and it wasn't a decision I took lightly. Though I had gone out of my way to spend time with children in the past—working at summer camps, volunteering in the nursery at church, spending time with nieces and nephews—having a child myself was a whole different thing. My struggles with illness would make raising kids incredibly challenging, and I preferred remaining childless.

"I know the expected answer is usually a resounding yes," I hastily added.

"Not always," Jordan replied. He told me that he was on my side of the fence (albeit closer to the fence than I was) in regard to having children. My answer was not a deal breaker.

A tsunami of relief rushed through my body, followed by a torrent of incredulity. It was too good to be true. What if he was just saying that because he liked me and didn't want to break up? Or, even if he was being honest, what if he changed his mind later? What if he only *thought* he was okay with it now, but when we were past the honeymoon stage, he realized that children were his dream? Was I being selfish by dating him?

Now, you know this story ends (or, rather, begins) happily with a wedding, but I'll explain how we got there.

DOCTOR WHO'S GUIDE TO COMMUNICATION

In the first episode of *Doctor Who*'s seventh series, Amy Pond finds herself expressing similar doubts about her husband and their capacity to have children. However, her situation is slightly different because she knows Rory definitely wants children. At the beginning of the episode, the two are headed for divorce—a shocking revelation for viewers like me who thought nothing could separate them. After all, Rory waited almost 2,000 years for her in Series Five, a fact he reminds her of in this episode:

"Amy, basic fact of our relationship is that I love you more than you love me," he says, adding that she was the one to kick him out.

In response, she slaps him. Because her love for him had never dwindled. She had, it turns out, signed the divorce papers out of love, in an effort to give Rory what he had always wanted:

"You want kids. You have always wanted kids, ever since you *were* a kid," she says. "And I can't have them … I can't ever give you children. I didn't kick you out. I gave you up."[2]

After this conversation, the tension between them dissipates. At the conclusion of the episode's pulse-racing adventure, the Doctor drops them off at their home, where they stand together on the sidewalk and share a look. Amy walks toward the house, and Rory correctly interprets her body language as an invitation to come in, so he does a little dance before following her. The subtext: their relationship has been mended now that the truth has come out. Their fears have been voiced; Amy was afraid that Rory would not want to be with her since she couldn't have children. Rory was afraid that Amy didn't love him as much as he loved her. Both fears were unfounded.

I don't know if anything could keep Rory from Amy after he realizes she still loves him. And that's his choice. Amy made the mistake of making the decision for him without giving him a say in the matter. She thought she knew best. She thought she was being selfless and loving; at least, that's probably what she told herself, even though fear spurred her choice. But it is Rory who gets to choose whether he wants to be with her or not. It is Rory who gets to choose whether children are a deal breaker for him or not.

Similarly, Jordan gets his own say in the matter, too. I have to trust that he can make his own decisions, and I don't have the right to assume I know what's "best" for him. He deserves my honesty. If he thinks his life is going to be more fulfilling *with* me and *without* kids, who am I to refuse him when I want to (and will) spend the rest of my life with him, too?

CHILDREN ARE EXPECTED

Deciding whether or not to have children is huge. It involves human lives—yours, an unborn baby's, and possibly a partner's. Often, there's added pressure because the expectation to have kids is everywhere, even in our beloved pop culture.

For example, In *Jurassic World*, Claire tells her sister she's unlikely to have children, and her sister insists that she will, telling her it's worth it. In *The Big Bang Theory*, Howard almost breaks up with Bernadette because she doesn't want kids; after they're married, Bernadette changes her mind, and they have a child together. Robin in *How I Met Your Mother* openly dislikes kids and doesn't want them. But, when she finds out she is physically incapable of having them, she's distraught by the news. These stories perpetuate the idea that women don't *really* know what they're saying when they voice their disinterest in having children.

Lifestyle blogger Jenny Mustard posted a video[3] in 2016 on her YouTube page about why she didn't want children. She cited minimalism, environmentalism, lifestyle, and simply not enjoying spending time with kids as her reasons. Among the 4,000-plus comments (many by women saying they're thankful they're not alone in the stigma they've faced for remaining childless) are statements that criticize her for her decision—that she must be saying she has bad genes if she doesn't want children; that she'd understand the value of children when she's eighty, frail, and dependent; that she shouldn't have a partner if she doesn't want kids; and that she's calling all children parasites.

There's a lot of judgment surrounding this decision—just ask a pregnant woman about all the unsolicited advice she receives on a daily basis. The assumption that family planning is fair game for public speculation is damaging. There are a thousand reasons why this is a personal topic, and bringing it up could cause unnecessary stress. One of my friends miscarried, and when she was picking up her daughter from child care, someone commented, "Oh, she doesn't want to go home because she has no one to play with." They were unaware of the miscarriage and no doubt felt it was an innocent comment. Instead, it just reminded my friend of the baby she lost—a reminder she certainly did not need.

In addition, many people think it's their job to speak up when a couple has decided *not* to have children.

My husband and I were setting up a joint account at our bank a few months after our wedding, and the associate (whom neither of us had met before) asked polite questions about our wedding. Then, she said, "So… having kids is next!"

I sat in stony silence, because she was not the first stranger to ask that question, and it irks me for so many reasons. What if I was infertile but desperately wanted children, and this question brought up difficult emotions? What if we were already trying and nervous about it? What if we *were* pregnant and hadn't told anyone yet and didn't want the first person we tell to be a random bank teller? What if we were in the midst of discussing children, hadn't come to a decision yet, and didn't want to get into it with a stranger? (Though I really do advise talking about that before you get married.) What if we didn't want kids and felt constantly judged?

What if it was a personal question and *none of your business*?

"No, we're not having kids," my husband replied.

"Ah," she said, nodding. "Not yet."

Not yet.

Ugh. Why would anyone think that is an appropriate thing to say? Jordan told her we were not having children, and she assumed we either didn't really know what we were talking about and would change our minds later, or that what he really meant was we weren't planning to have children in the immediate future.

I shouldn't have to defend myself to people asking, "Why aren't you having kids?" It's not a question you ask about people who *are* having children. "So, why *are* you having kids?" just sounds plain rude. But people continue to ask me, often on top of saying other inappropriate things, like "You'll change your mind one day," "You won't understand what real love is until you hold your own child in your arms," or "You'd be much more fulfilled if you had children."

FYI, I have no problem with close friends and family asking me personal questions, including ones about family planning. They have a relationship with me. They're allowed. It's strangers and acquaintances forcing their opinions on me that weirds me out.

The conservative Christian culture I grew up in is especially bad for this, where women who are childless by choice are attacked for not reading their Bible correctly and not following God's purpose for their lives (i.e., to "be fruitful and multiply"). Others simply think it's selfish to avoid procreation. I often don't have the energy to explain my reasoning, and I don't always want to go into the details of my chronic illness every time I'm asked this inappropriate question by strangers.

In an online article on *Refinery29*, Britney Gil writes about the abuse she'd experienced from her father and her reasons for remaining childless:

> "I have often heard people claim that not having children is selfish—that it's a shirking of responsibility, based on petty desires to be comfortable and travel and sleep late on weekends. But mine is a choice between two possible outcomes: That I may have children and regret it, or that I may not have children and regret it. The latter would certainly be sad, a decision that I could never take back. But the first impacts another human being for the rest of their life, and the second impacts only me. If making the second choice is selfish, then I must be using a different definition of the term."[4]

Unfortunately, people will always say the wrong thing. I'm as guilty of doing it as the next person. I can let myself get riled up every time it happens, or I can take a deep breath and move on with my life. If I've come to a point of acceptance about my condition and choices, it's easier to let others' inappropriate remarks go. While they may still spark feelings of guilt, shame, sadness, or anger, it's easier to focus on the people who accept my decision than the ones who don't.

While our culture screams at us that having children is expected, the norm, the *mandatory*—maybe it's not. Maybe it's something we should deeply consider. Maybe we should be asking questions like "Why do I want (or not want) children?" and "How will this impact the lives involved?" And for those of us struggling with chronic illnesses, "How will having a child impact my illness, and how will my illness impact my child?"

FACTORING IN CHRONIC ILLNESS

Those of us with chronic pain think twice about having children because we already have trouble taking care of ourselves, never mind someone else.

As a young adult, I didn't pause to consider why I might *not* want children. I didn't realize *married and childless* was an option. I liked the idea of being a stay-at-home mom because I liked the stay-at-home part. I had no idea that being a parent was a 24/7 job with no sick days and no time off. In more recent years, seeing many of my friends courageously and lovingly embrace parenthood opened my eyes to how much energy goes into making sure these little people flourish.

It has also made me ask myself whether I could handle being a parent. Would pregnancy be too difficult on my body? And after the child was born, would I be able to manage a living, breathing person who needed me to stay alive? When I already don't get enough sleep, would I be able to stay sane after being up with a baby all night?

Due to my illness, I would not be able to give my child the amount of attention I'd want. I would miss important milestones in her life due to IBS attacks at inopportune times. I would be an exhausted, depressed, unhealthy mess.

I also cringe at the thought of passing on my condition to a child. IBS seems to be genetic; my mom has it and so do several grandparents. It would be tough seeing my kid going through the same amount of pain that I experience. This is an issue for many with chronic diseases—what if we pass them on? No loving parent wants to see their child in pain and endure the guilt of choosing to have a child despite knowing an inherited illness is likely.

None of these "what if" fears are reasons to avoid having children, especially if having kids is your dream. They are just potential difficulties that people with chronic illnesses think about. Since I don't have a burning desire to be a mom, remaining childless is the best decision for me. Others may decide differently, based on their particular illness, circumstances, or a partner's desire and willingness to stay at home to raise the child(ren).

"I've thought about not having kids due to my migraines, which are often debilitating," says Joy Beth Smith, a thirty-one-year-old editor and the author of *Party of One: Truth, Longing, and the Subtle Art of Singleness*:

"I grew up with a mom who had migraines, so I know the neglect that comes from this set-up; the pain truly is unbearable, and if I'm getting sick, I have no other option but to lie down in a dark, cold room. What would I do if I had children, much less a baby? What if I was a single mom? My own single mother made choices I'd like to think I wouldn't, but who's to say. When you're in that much pain several days a month, or a migraine that lingers for several days, and that situation is compounded by the stress of motherhood, you are desperate."

Joy Beth says the choice to have children would probably depend on her future husband's desire to have kids and his own availability. "If I was married to a man who wasn't passionate about kids, I would never want to bear the lion's share of that on my own, combined with the weight of a marriage," she says. "I'd be content to find a non-profit to volunteer at and spoil the malarkey out of my nieces."

As Joy Beth points out, there are other ways to fill your life with children even if you don't have them yourself. This is not necessarily a consolation for those who badly want children of their own and can't have them, just a fact for those who judge childless people too quickly.

PARENTING WITH A CHRONIC ILLNESS

Many with chronic illnesses are willing to make the sacrifices involved in raising a child and choose to do so (hopefully with a fabulous support system to help). For others, the illness occurs after they are already parents. In either case, family may not look the way they hoped or expected due to illness. Parents with chronic illness face some incredible challenges on top of the already challenging aspects of parenting. These can include:

- Learning to put your needs ahead of your child's and partner's sometimes to avoid burnout. It's intuitive that children come first, but destroying yourself in the process isn't doing them any favours.
- Asking for help.
- Managing fatigue.
- Trying not to dwell on questions like "What if it gets worse?"
- Changing expectations of what your family life looks like. Your children may not be able to do all the extracurricular activities they (or you) want, your house may not be clean most of the time, the dishes may pile up, you may need to rely on others, and so on.
- Dealing with mental health struggles.
- Revising your plans to have more children.
- Explaining to your child why you're so tired, sick, or in pain a lot of the time.
- Disappointing your child because you can't always do what they want. Being patient with their emotional responses is difficult when you're also frustrated with your limits.
- Helping them come to terms with your illness. They may experience fear at the thought of losing you or seeing you in pain. They may even

> feel guilty and wonder if it's their fault or if they
> are exacerbating your symptoms.

After having cancer as a child, Sara, a forty-two-year-old wife and mother, has a host of health problems. She is proud of her age because it's a victory she has lived this long.

Due to the side effects from a blood transfusion, she had Hepatitis C until 2004. Due to side effects from chemo and radiation, she currently has muscle degradation that can make moving around uncomfortable, heart issues including cardiomyopathy (she will one day need a heart transplant), and a compromised immune system—plus, she is unable to have children.

Sara and her husband decided to adopt. They have two children, a twelve-year-old named Zoe and a three-year-old they refer to as Little Dude on social media because of fostering privacy. "We thought three children at least… but that has changed," she says.

Since her body is being attacked on so many fronts, she doesn't have the energy to keep up with them as much as she would like, never mind keeping the house tidy and getting household chores done in a reasonable time. She gives the kids more screen time than she would like so she can rest and leans on family members to help out.

> "I wasn't allowed to pick up Zoe after she turned two, because I was at risk for a heart attack," Sara recalls. "Try dealing with a tantrum from a cold toddler who doesn't want to leave the park, but it's February and you need to get the two of you home, and you can't just pick the kid

up to make her leave. It was the last time we went to the park until winter was over."

She also points out that kids spread germs with fervour, which makes it difficult for her immune system. She gets lots of colds and flus and has to get the pneumonia vaccine because the virus can kill someone with heart failure. If she *does* get pneumonia, one of the few antibiotics that work for her can also hurt someone with heart issues.

Sara worries about how much to tell her children about her health. She doesn't want to scare Zoe, but she also doesn't want to surprise her with a health concern and have her wondering what she's hiding the rest of the time. She feels terrible when the children have to see her in the hospital, because they miss her and are scared.

"Little Dude doesn't understand a whole lot of it," she says. "He begs to have me pick him up, and I can't."

Sara hadn't expected parenting to be this difficult. When she and her husband, Jason, first decided to adopt, they thought the worst of her health issues were over. It had been a decade since she had cancer, the Hepatitis C was gone, and they hadn't expected any more side effects from the chemo or radiation until the symptoms hit her. But Sara had always wanted to be a mother, so they adopted Zoe. And when Zoe's brother was in need of foster care, she couldn't say no:

"Having the siblings grow up together is so valuable. I knew it would be hard. Jason knew it would mean a lot of sacrifice on his part because a lot more of the weight of parenting would fall on him."

Although Sara and Jason have decided not to add more

children to their family, Sara says that parenting has provided her with a purpose unlike anything else in her life.

"I'm still not sure that saying yes to our Little Dude was the right choice for me. [But was it] the right choice for him, for my husband, for Zoe, for many other people involved in his life? YES indeed!" she says. "This is it for me, though. I might occasionally babysit grandkids in the future, but I'll certainly never be the kind of grandma that does the full-time childcare while their parents are at work! Which is assuming I live that long. Longevity is always an unknown... even for people with healthy bodies."

Parenting is a full-time job. So is having a chronic illness. Taking on one or both are acts of heroism that rival the Doctor's. Whether you decide to have children, choose to remain childless, or have the decision taken from you, you're not selfish for taking your illness into account. Fear is the biggest barrier when it comes to family plans because, like Amy Pond, we get caught up in what other people think of us. We get scared that we're being selfish, and we wonder if our illness will make things impossible. But in the end, we make the choices we can with the circumstances we're in. We make space for our illnesses and ask others to do the same. We reap joy from the children in our lives, whether they're ours or someone else's, and we accept when our lives look different than others'.

9

WOMEN. SEX. THE MOON.

"Dear me. Ladies. God bless 'em. What would we do without them... with their ways... their mysterious seasons... the moon... Glenn Close... Sheena Easton... all the different kinds of women. Smashing!"[1]

— MAURICE MOSS, *THE IT CROWD*

*W*hen it's 10:00 p.m. but your pee starts to feel like acid and your bladder like it might explode, you go to the ER.

I was pretty lucid as I checked in with the nurse. Though I have a high pain tolerance, that doesn't mean I experience pain less, it just means I don't necessarily show it on my face. I told her I was in a lot of pain, and she typed something into the computer with a bored expression on her face. I then proceeded to sit down in the waiting room with my husband, and we waited. And waited.

Women suffering from chronic pain are frequently

told they have a mental condition and are misdiagnosed with depression or anxiety. It can take several years (and seeing several specialists) to receive an accurate diagnosis and appropriate standard of care.[2] There's also a cycle of bias that occurs when women report pain in the emergency room or doctor's office. That night, I experienced it first-hand.

Hours passed as I started peeing blood and the pain increased. I approached the nurse again, this time unable to control the tears in my eyes. She said the only thing she could do was give me some Advil, which I declined at first.

After a few minutes, I went back to the nurse and took her up on the offer because, even though I was certain my pain was too advanced for an Advil to help, I had to do something. She showed no empathy. No sympathy. I felt judged. I feared she thought I was crying on purpose simply to get in to see a doctor quicker; either that or she assumed I was a hysterical female and wasn't actually in that much pain.

My only options to demonstrate my pain levels were to attempt stoicism, in which case she didn't believe I was in that much pain, or to show more emotion, in which case she wrote me off as overly emotional. There was no right answer.

I couldn't help contrasting my experience with my husband's. When we rushed him to the ER because of intense abdominal pain, the nurse immediately offered him a Tylenol 3 (a much stronger pain reliever) while we waited. I wondered why they hadn't extended the same courtesy to me when my symptoms looked much the same as his had. Though my pain was just as intense and lasted longer, the only thing I was offered was Advil. This contrasting experience mirrors the results of a 2008 study that found women were less likely to receive opiates (a more effective type of pain relievers) for their pain than men.[3]

"Since women are expected to have an overly emotional response to pain, they are at risk of having their reports not taken seriously whether they adhere to the stereotype or break with it," writes Maya Dusenbery in her book *Doing Harm*. "Conversely, the expectation that men keep a stiff upper lip when they're in pain serves to ensure that they're likely to be taken seriously no matter what: if they're stoic, they're just being a typical 'macho' guy, and if they're emotional, well, then it must be really, really bad."[4]

Though we arrived at the ER around 11:00 p.m., I didn't get to see a doctor until 9:00 a.m., a full ten hours later. It was ten hours of agonizing, non-stop pain. I still experience anxiety when I recall that trip to the ER. I can't help but wonder if I would have gotten in sooner, or even if the nurse would have offered me more empathy (and a Tylenol 3), if I were a man.

MEN AND SEX

In *Ask Me about My Uterus*, Abby Norman writes about the long journey it took before she finally discovered she had endometriosis, a painful condition where tissue that normally lines the uterus grows outside of it (though this is a simplified definition as there are cases of men with endometriosis). Abby details a life where she was repeatedly hospitalized due to intense abdominal pain, and doctors continually misdiagnosed her and told her the symptoms were psychological. It took her boyfriend accompanying her to a doctor's appointment complaining that their sex life was being affected before she was taken seriously. She writes:

"Once I started taking Max with me to appointments, and he corroborated—or better yet, expressed his own frustration—suddenly it seemed like doctors started to listen... It either meant that they hadn't believed me in the absence of Max as an alibi, or that they had believed me, but my suffering alone wasn't enough to inspire action. Becoming a disappointment to a man, though, seemed to do the trick."[5]

The cringe-worthy descriptions of the pain she went through and my desire for these stigmas to disappear are difficult to handle. Every time Abby writes about another professional who doesn't believe her, I wince. She also details feeling guilty about being unable to satisfy her boyfriend's sexual desires, and feeling frustrated that her own desires were obstructed by pain.

This was a deep fear I faced in the first few months of my marriage—that my husband would lose interest in me or love me less because of the undiagnosed condition that causes me pain during intercourse.

I felt guilty when we avoided sex because it was too painful. I debated just doing it anyway, and might have lived through months of painful sex if my husband hadn't verbally confirmed he didn't want to cause me pain.

Abby writes that Max, her boyfriend, took the rejection personally. "Of course, my sexual needs weren't being met either, but no one really asked me if I was sexually frustrated."[6]

Eventually, Max became so embittered that he told her it was only fair that he sleep with other women. Yes, you read that right. In her book, Abby relates her struggle with shame and her attempt to understand his perspective. She was working so hard to accommodate him, to keep him happy, she couldn't focus on what she needed.

Many women who are diagnosed with chronic illnesses after heterosexual marriage face challenges from their husbands' attitudes. Men are often sympathetic at first, but less so as time wears on. They begin to resent their wives for not having the energy to cook, clean, or take care of their children.

According to a 2009 study, a woman diagnosed with a serious medical illness is six times more likely to be left by her partner than a man with the same illness.[7] Weirdly enough, one of the reasons for this may be fear of abandonment—men typically rely on their spouses for emotional support, and when there's a threat of that support disappearing, they leave sooner so they don't have to suffer the pain of losing her later. I don't get it. But, then again, I'm a woman.

Marital expectations are at play here as well—assuming a wife will fulfill a specific role (perhaps the traditional one of caregiver, mom, cook, and maid) and feeling lost when she's not emotionally available, the kids need someone else to look after them, dinner isn't on the table, and the bathtub scum may come alive at any moment.

That many men feel like they're owed this type of labour is the fault of a society that tells them so, and I wish more men were brought up like my husband with the understanding that women are equals.

It's frustrating that so little research goes into female health issues. It's inexcusable that my body is considered less important than a male's.

FEMALE PAIN IS EXPECTED

Sara Jane has had fibromyalgia for about ten years. Fibromyalgia is an under-researched disorder where you experience widespread pain and exhaustion. She describes everything hurting, a lack of energy, weakness, feeling like her tongue is scalded, extreme sensitivity to touch, pain during sex, blurry vision, and brain fog. Women are more likely to develop fibromyalgia than men.

Her doctor misdiagnosed her with anxiety. She says, "He just sent me out the door to deal with it." Through investigations of her own and the discovery that fibromyalgia runs in her family, Sara Jane finally figured out the name of her condition.

She describes coming to terms with her illness and her frustration with it, accepting she can't do the things she used to, and learning to say no without feeling guilty that she's letting people down. She adds that it took her much longer to get over her anger about the differences between men and women and how she's suffered as a female.

"I've run into barriers all my life because of things I want to do," she says, listing leadership in church, sports, and other male-dominated activities. "I also had sexual dysfunction problems that are female. And I thought, this isn't fair. Why don't I get to enjoy this the way men do? The whole realm of sexual pleasure is completely different for women than men, but I wasn't taught a thing about it."

I was nodding along as Sara Jane spoke because I wasn't taught much about sex either. A few months before my wedding, one of my friends sent me a link to an article from *The Week* titled, "The female price of male pleasure." She mentioned that she didn't have a lot of sexual knowledge before getting married, and the information would have been useful for her to know back then. Written by Lili Loofbourow, the article explains why "the world is disturbingly comfortable with the fact that women sometimes leave a sexual encounter in tears."[8] Lili writes that women are enculturated to accept pain and discomfort for the sake of male pleasure, and many don't say anything when sex hurts.

According to a 2018 clinical review on female sexual pain published in *Cureus*, "Women suffering from dyspareunia [pain during sex] may struggle to find support and acknowledgement that their pain is 'real.' Many women report being dismissed and invalidated."[9]

As I read these articles, I thought, *But sex is supposed to hurt. At least, for the first time. And maybe for a while after. But then it gets better, right?*

Unfortunately, this question wasn't hypothetical for me. Due to an as-yet undiagnosed condition, sex hurts for me, like I'm being stabbed from the inside out.[10] When this happened the first time, guess what my reaction was?

It was to say nothing. To get it over with.

But when my husband asked me if I was okay, I couldn't lie to him. When I said it hurt, he immediately stopped. And that action, my friends, is an example of someone who has questioned societal norms and does not consider his pleasure worth someone else's pain. For his consideration of my comfort, I am incredibly grateful.

I spent a large part of the rest of the night in tears—not because of the pain, but because I felt ashamed I couldn't provide the pleasure that was supposed to happen on a wedding night. Jordan held me and told me it was okay, that he hadn't married me in order to have sex. Thank goodness for that. We've both since learned that Hollywood's portrayal of marriage and sex is nothing like reality—sex can be wonderful, and physical intimacy is important in a marriage, but there are a variety of ways to be intimate. Sex should be enjoyable for both people, and if it's causing one partner to be in pain, they're well within their rights to say "slow down" or to stop the activity altogether.

It's taken patience and experimentation to figure out how to have sex comfortably. And I'm not unique in my struggles. Inflammation, infection, endometriosis, STIs, pelvic inflammatory disease, cystitis, ovarian cysts, and many other conditions can cause pain during sex (I know, because I've been tested for most of them), not to mention psychological issues and stress that can affect the body, causing muscles to tighten and sex to be uncomfortable or painful as a result.

It makes a world of difference when committed sexual partners are understanding instead of presumptuous, when they don't assume male pleasure is worth the price of female pain. Pain is not something women just need to get over. We're allowed to say no, to search for solutions to our discomfort, to avoid suffering when we have a choice.

WOMEN'S HEALTH IS A BLOODY MESS. PERIOD.

When Sara Jane told me her frustrations about being a woman, she also mentioned having incredibly painful periods. She recalls having to leave class during her first year of college because the pain was so bad. She sat in the bathroom, moaning and groaning, wondering how she would make it back to her dorm. "I was in so much pain," she says, "I imagined headlines: 'Girl dies of menstrual cramps.'"

If you're thinking, *Wow. Melodramatic much?* then you are one of the lucky people who has not had to call in sick for work or stayed home from school because you could barely move due to the intense pain coursing through your stomach—pain caused by this "normal" bodily function. Some women have it easier, with mild twinges and a penny's worth of blood to deal with. Others, like Sara Jane and me, experience incredible pain and torrents of blood that can rush out on cue at a single sneeze. Sometimes the cramps trigger my IBS, too—double cramp attacks. Yay. Painful periods add another layer of stress and discomfort to women dealing with chronic pain.

There's an episode of one of my favourite comedies, *The IT Crowd*, in which Jen gets her "time of the month" and hilarity ensues due to her ignorant male co-workers, Roy and Moss. The two men are confused and frightened when she suddenly yells at them and literally turns into a she-devil for a few seconds.

Eventually, Roy and Moss also start acting irritable, yelling at each other and throwing a computer onto the floor, so Jen asks them what's wrong:

Jen: What on earth is going on?
Moss: I dunno, I feel weird. And I've been swearing like a flippin' docker.
Roy: Denholm just thanked me… and I started crying like an actress... I feel delicate. And, um, annoyed. And, um, I think I'm ugly.[11]

Jen hypothesizes that the two men somehow "synced up" with her cycle the way her previous female roommates used to, and they spend the rest of the episode attempting to deal with their rampant emotions (while sharing a hot water bottle to ease stomach cramps).

Though Roy and Moss are unable to empathize with Jen at the beginning, they are much more patient after they have experienced some of her symptoms themselves. I've no doubt the stigma surrounding periods, and women's pain in general, would disappear if men experienced these things too. But I'll settle for men attempting to understand and advocating for our health.

I recently read a social media thread where men admitted misconceptions they'd had about periods, such as believing that menstrual bleeding can only happen during the day. Women also detailed their encounters with male confusion, such as having to explain to a boss that they really did have to leave a meeting so they could put on a tampon and avoid bleeding onto the chair; no, they couldn't just "hold it in." A surprising number of men believed that women could just pee out their blood when they wanted and didn't understand why tampons or pads were necessary.

This lack of knowledge and these misconceptions are mirrored in women's health in general. A 2018 study found that doctors misdiagnose heart attacks in women more than they do men, because the symptoms in women are different than in men.[12]

A lot of the research that has been done to differentiate between male and female responses hasn't been fully integrated into medical education, which is why so many doctors are unaware of these differences.

PubMed lists about five times more clinical trials focusing on erectile dysfunction than dyspareunia, vaginismus, and vulvodynia combined. Women are more likely to experience side effects from drugs because they've mainly been tested on men. Women are under-represented in many research areas, and when they are included, researchers don't necessarily analyze their findings by sex or gender.

Women's pain matters. We need more representation in the medical community and more people listening when we are suffering.

MAKING PEACE WITH BEING FEMALE

I'm proud of being a woman. I'm proud of how far we've come. I'm thankful for the women, men, and non-binary people who are allies and advocates.

I'm also frustrated with being a woman. I'm frustrated that we still have so far to go, that men still think I'm worth less than they are, that I have to fight to be considered equal. I'm also frustrated because, with my health issues, I often don't have the energy to fight. I sit in the ER for ten hours while people who are in less pain get in to see a doctor ahead of me, and I do nothing because I am in too much pain to move. I feel helpless to change the system. While I don't want to force men (or anyone else) to experience my periods or chronic illnesses, it's frustrating that pain is what it would take for many to sit up and listen.

I don't accept things the way they are, but I accept that I am doing what I can to change them, that my voice matters, that even though I often feel useless, I matter. I don't understand why society works this way or why female bodies work this way, but I know it's not all in my head and I'm not alone. If Moss and Roy can learn to empathize with a woman, surely others can too.

10

FUEL FOR ANXIETY

"It makes it hard to not be scared all the time."[1]

— AMANDA BROTZMAN, *DIRK GENTLY'S*
HOLISTIC DETECTIVE AGENCY

I'm afraid of pain and that it might never go away. I'm afraid of being a burden. I'm afraid doctors won't listen to me and will, instead, discredit my experiences. I'm afraid of tests and side effects. I'm afraid friends will get tired of me. I'm afraid my husband will acclimatize to my illness and become less sympathetic over time. I'm afraid to leave the house. I'm afraid that, during a simple chore like grocery shopping, I'll have to sit down in the middle of the aisle due to a wave of nausea and people will stare (yes, this has happened to me).

Amanda Brotzman, a character from Hulu's *Dirk Gently's Holistic Detective Agency*, spent years as a shut-in prior to the beginning of the series. Amanda has pararibulitis, a fictional disease where she experiences hallucinations that feel real. As her brother Todd describes, "Water on your hand could feel like fire. Your shoe on your foot could feel like it was crushing it. Breathing could feel like drowning."[2] Yikes.

When Todd visits her in Episode One, "Horizons," the two of them jam together—Amanda on the drums and Todd on the guitar. But in the middle of rocking out, Amanda suddenly perceives one of her drumsticks as a knife slicing into her hand. She jumps up, screaming from the pain as Todd tries to calm her.

Amanda rarely leaves the house due to anxiety. However, when Dirk Gently learns of her illness, he asks her why she never goes out. "If the disease is in you, why does it matter where you go?" he asks her. These are innocent words from someone who has never experienced the kind of anxiety Amanda has. I would probably have been offended and tried to explain what it was like living with an illness, but Amanda just looks at him in surprise, as if she's never thought of it that way. It is, no doubt, these words that inspire her to make a trip to the grocery store all by herself in Episode Three.

It's just a short scene—a small moment you might miss if you are unfamiliar with the fear a chronic illness can inspire. Amanda walks down a grocery store aisle with a shopping basket in her hand, struggling to breathe through the anxiety. As she picks up a cheese sample and tastes it, her expression slowly shifts from panic to delight. I suspect she is thinking something like, *I'm out of the house, and I'm not having an attack. I'm okay. I can do this.* She slams the basket down on the checkout counter in victory and tells the confused cashier, "I made it." She is so proud of herself, delighted with the freedom of doing something on her own.

And then her hand is engulfed in fire—flames only she can see and feel. She struggles to open her pill bottle and spills her medication onto the floor, screaming. She races into the parking lot and collapses, feeling fire engulf her body and burn her flesh, as two guys laugh at her and record the whole thing with their phones.

Her anxiety seeps into me as I watch this scene, and I feel her relief as the Rowdy Three, a strange group of characters with mystical abilities, race to her rescue, chase off the gogglers, and magically feed off of her anxiety, which gives her a reprieve from the pain.

THE DESIRE FOR SELF-SUFFICIENCY

Most North Americans expect self-sufficiency. The whole "pull yourself up by your bootstraps" thing is like a religion. Adults who live with their parents, or who can't change a flat tire, or who've never done their own taxes are the butts of jokes. People who can't seem to keep a job are frowned upon. *What's wrong with them?* we ask, even though there is often nothing wrong with *them*—stuff just happens, and it's beyond people's control.

I know exactly what's wrong with me. Because I'm super sick, I can't always do everything for myself. But I want to so badly. I hate asking other people to do things for me. I want to be perceived as strong and self-reliant and gets-things-done. I want to be able to go to the grocery store, the library, the drugstore, the bank, get a haircut, get work done, make supper, and visit friends all in one day. But often, all I can manage is one of those things, and my husband, family member, or friend helps with the rest, or the rest waits for another day.

One morning, I woke up early with an attack of cramps, and I proceeded to the bathroom with a book to hopefully distract me from the pain. However, the pain increased at an exponential level, and I called Jordan from the bedroom to come stand beside me so I could lean on him. In addition to the volcano erupting in my gut, I felt woozy and nauseated, but I couldn't leave the toilet because my bowels threatened to let loose at any moment. I was covered in sweat and even uttering a single word took massive effort. My vision darkened. The pain exploded, and I felt like I was dying; I would cease to exist if it increased anymore.

The next thing I remember, I was awakening to Jordan holding me up; my book was on the floor, the pages crumpled. I had passed out. I was delirious and confused at first, like waking up from a nightmare. The pain gradually eased up from there, and I was able to retreat to the bed. Then I began shaking and shivering, even under the blanket and with Jordan's body heat next to me. I don't know if this intense cold is my body overcompensating after overheating or if it's because I'm in shock after the intense pain, but it always happens after a severe attack.

I'm almost always anxious about leaving the house, but after attacks like this, that anxiety is increased a hundred-fold. It's scary not knowing when you will be in intense pain, or, when you are in the midst of it, not knowing how long it will last. You can get post-traumatic stress and anxiety from the intense experiences of pain itself and from the fear those memories of pain incur.

A week after this episode, I would get panic attacks

simply from leaving the house, even in the company of my husband. After about a week being confined to our little condo, I realized my anxiety about leaving might not get better until I left. So I went out with my husband for an hour. I panicked, but I survived. After experiences like these, it's important to celebrate small victories. This was victory number one.

A few days later, I decided to go grocery shopping on my own. I didn't *feel* brave enough. But I did it anyway. I felt like Amanda, walking down the aisles, worried I would experience an attack, of pain, nausea, or anxiety, at any moment.

I felt a twinge in my stomach, and anxiety shot through me, flooding my system with panic. I stopped, leaning against the cart, and breathed. In. Out. In. Out. Suddenly I was submersed in an ocean of nausea. Great.

In. Out. In. Out. One step forward, and then the next. I finished grabbing the items from my list and made it to the checkout. I got to my car with the groceries. I made it home. Victory number two.

A week after that, I was able to drive to a music rehearsal without feeling any anxiety at all. Victory number three.

Managing my anxiety is a balancing act; I have to decide every day what my limits are, when to push myself, and when to give myself a break.

"THERE'S A CONCEPT CALLED PAIN ANXIETY," says Dr. Jason Ediger, a psychologist in Winnipeg, Manitoba. "The more afraid we are of our pain, the more we experience subjective pain and the more disruptive that pain is to our lives."

Jason recommends pacing techniques, acceptance therapy, and mindfulness-based approaches as viable ways to cope long-term with unsolvable and unpredictable pain. Pacing techniques are about finding the middle road between using up too much energy and avoiding life altogether. Acceptance and mindfulness are about acknowledging the reality of pain and our inability to control it.

"I've had some patients who got good results greeting the pain that would show up in random attacks," he says. "For example, 'Hey, there you are. Where have you been all morning?'—then moving back to the task at hand."

My anxiety hasn't disappeared. I haven't "conquered" it, which is an unrealistic goal anyway. I'm learning to manage it, and that's enough. I don't always decide to be brave. Sometimes, the anxiety and stress on my body is just not worth it, and I make the decision to stay home. Choosing to stay home and miss an event, meeting, appointment, or outing is not "losing the battle"; it's managing a condition. And sometimes this is the braver decision of the two.

I've learned to give myself compassion and grace. I have a "fight it and conquer it" mentality, and I feel guilty when my condition persists. All my favourite stories from pop culture are about battling and defeating evil. And sickness sure seems evil to me.

I've been especially angry at myself for not being able to conquer the mental health issues that spiral out of control due to illness. Depression and anxiety—those are all in my head. They're not "real" issues like a broken limb or a paralyzed body, so I should be able to fix them if I just concentrate hard enough, right?

Since Albus Dumbledore is a paragon of wisdom, it stands to reason he'd have a quote to fit this situation, and he does: "Of course it is happening inside your head, Harry, but why on earth should that mean it is not real?"[3] A tattoo-worthy quote if there ever was one.

Despite the light recently being shed on mental health conditions, there's still a stigma associated with them. Sometimes, that stigma comes from the very people who suffer from the conditions. Sometimes, it comes from me.

DON'T CONTRIBUTE TO THE STIGMA

"I'm sorry," I said to my friend as we found an empty bench in the crowded mall to sit down on. I had become overwhelmed, felt that chest-tightening panic blooming like a corpse flower, and needed to take a break from shopping for a moment. My stomach was also retaliating, of course, and I made sure the spot was near the bathroom in case I needed to make a break for it.

"Don't apologize! It's no problem!" she replied, because she's awesome.

My anxiety is not my fault. It's nothing I need to apologize for, and yet I still feel the need to. I feel bad I'm inconveniencing people.

"What's wrong with me? Why can't I just get over it?" I ask myself. Those are useless, unhelpful questions. There are so many factors that contribute to anxiety—genetics, environment, neurology, trauma.

Anxiety about getting sick isn't illogical either, because I will absolutely have another attack. Sometime. Somewhere. It's going to happen. It'll be painful and inconvenient and horrible. The anxiety in anticipation of this event doesn't *help*, of course. When I experience cramping and wonder if it'll pass or get worse, when the dread tightens my muscles, it can actually increase the fire in my stomach.

When I treat these panic attacks as my fault, when I do things like apologize to people because of them, I'm only contributing to an abusive perspective of mental health.

People develop behaviours that make anxiety worse, such as making unhealthy choices, avoiding everything, destroying support systems, or encouraging negative thought patterns, but these are coping mechanisms *because* of anxiety. New, healthy methods of coping can be learned. The methods you've used to survive don't mean you are a horrible person or have anything to apologize for.

The only thing I am to blame for is contributing to a stigma that already exists by treating myself badly.

ANXIETY ATTACKS

I didn't understand the difference between anxiety and depression, or that anxiety wasn't just about "worrying too much," until I had a full-blown anxiety attack a few years ago. I lay in bed, my brain a game of *Tetris* in which random thoughts flew by too fast for me to fit together. Suddenly my chest tightened and my breathing quickened. I was lightheaded, and didn't understand what was going on. I felt scared, panicked, and alone.

Sometimes anxiety just hits me like that for no apparent reason. Other times, it's associated with leaving the house or being in an uncomfortable situation. The mere memory of anxiety attacks, doing so while writing this right now, makes breathing feel like a chore and my chest tighten up. I have to remind myself to relax and to take deep breaths. Sometimes, I fear the anxiety itself, and *that* makes me anxious. It's a vicious cycle.

People who have intense encounters with pain and anxiety can also have post-traumatic stress from the experiences. I've been hesitant to recognize this condition in myself because it is so often associated with life-threatening events, serious injuries, or sexual abuse, and I feel like a fraud for saying I have post-traumatic stress in my safe, sheltered environment.

In an article for *The Mighty*, Rachel Meeks writes, "My PTSD from chronic pain is very real, and actually makes a lot of sense. Why does calling a doctor put me in the throes of depression? Why have all my break-down-into-uncontrollable-crying episodes happened in hospitals? Perhaps my brain is perceiving doctors and hospitals as threats."[4]

She describes experiencing incredible stress when she has to phone or visit her doctor. And maybe that sounds illogical to a healthy person, but I know what she's talking about.

When you're sick, doctors are supposed to provide solutions, and for everyday, diagnosable illnesses, they usually do. But most people with chronic illnesses are sick all the time because there isn't a cure or because they haven't been properly diagnosed and doctors don't know how to fix them.

When a new symptom crops up and it merits a visit to

the doctor, I get incredibly nervous and stressed with thoughts like:

What if this is something my doctor can't fix and it's another thing I'll have to live with forever? What if she puts me on a medication with horrible side effects, like last time?

What if this results in more uncomfortable testing, like a colonoscopy or a pelvic exam?

What if she doesn't believe me or dismisses my pain as unimportant?

This anxiety increases tenfold if I'm going to see a *new* doctor or specialist that my GP has referred me to, because they are an unknown entity. At least I am relatively sure my GP will take me seriously, but I've had meetings with other specialists where they seem to think that, since they can't determine the cause of my pain, it either doesn't exist or I am exaggerating and it's really not that bad.

WHEN I WAS TWENTY-TWO, I saw a specialist after having a colonoscopy, who confirmed that I had irritable bowel syndrome (something I already knew but had never gotten the official diagnosis for). I felt completely brushed aside during the appointment, like he didn't believe me when I described my symptoms. He also referred to me as "fortunate" because I mentioned I have some periods of feeling okay interspersed with periods of sickness. *Lucky me, I'm only in incredible pain PART of the time!* He recommended I increase the fibre in my diet and then proceeded to dictate a letter to my GP about me as if I wasn't still sitting there in his office. I felt uncomfortable.

I wish all doctors had a magical bedside manner that exuded immediate waves of comfort and safety. Unfortunately, many of them do not. And many doctors have *never experienced chronic pain themselves.* This is important to note, because sometimes I just assume doctors should automatically know exactly what a patient is going through. A friend of a friend, who is a doctor, experienced chronic back pain after retirement. It was only then that he realized exactly what chronic pain felt like and expressed regrets about the way he treated past patients who came to him because of chronic pain.

It's difficult to be angry about doctors who don't understand when the problem is a lack of knowledge and ability to empathize rather than deliberate mistreatment. As much as I want to rail at doctors as being at fault for my anxiety, it's often not their fault. They can work to become more empathetic or sympathetic, but most are doing their jobs the best way they know how.

FINANCIAL ANXIETY

When Todd leaves Amanda's home in Episode One of *Dirk Gently*, he hands her a wad of cash. Amanda pockets it with a depressed look and quietly thanks him. Todd later explains to Dirk that it's for her medication, which she can't afford on her own. It's unclear how Amanda is able to afford housing when she doesn't have a job or how she gets by on her own, though it's implied Todd helps out a lot.

Often, the more sick you are, the more money you need—to have a place to live, to eat, to pay bills, and to afford medications, tests, and doctors. The problem is, the more sick you are, the less you're able to work. So how are you supposed to afford these things? What if you have a family to support? What if you're a lone parent with a child who's counting on you? Or what if you're single with no one to support you?

"I had to start freelancing and burned through almost all of my savings trying to keep up with treatments and survive while I tried to find enough work to stay afloat," says Elisabeth, a writer with Gilbert's disease. "Now, I'm too sick to work full-time (but not sick enough to go on disability, at least on paper) and am trying to scrape together enough income from my various part-time employments to survive."

I don't know what the process is in the United States or other countries, but qualifying for disability in Canada is more complicated than it may seem. Being too sick to work isn't all that's needed. Your illness has to be a recognized disability. In my case, irritable bowel syndrome is not one such illness. There are too many variations of it, and many people don't have it to the painful extent I do. I solved my work issues (mostly) by becoming self-employed and working from home. The stress of needing to be somewhere every day at a certain time can make chronic illness worse to live with. I might not actually be sick every day, but the constant fear that I will miss a meeting, be late, or inconvenience a co-worker is exhausting—never mind experiencing the pain itself.

During university, my parents helped me out a lot with finances. Afterward, I was single and constantly had just enough to make it through the month with my free-lance income. Living month to month is stressful. I like to plan for the future, and I like to be prepared. I'm thankful

I now have a husband who works full time; we can survive on his income alone, though I still feel guilty when I haven't done any freelance work to help contribute. I still have this desire to be self-sufficient. I have to remind myself I'm still valuable even if I'm not a money-making machine.

There is a particular type of financial anxiety I have not experienced to its fullest, thanks to my Canadian citizenship: wracking up thousands of dollars of debt in order to pay for medical tests. In general, my health care has been accessible and affordable, so I don't have to endure having a camera stuck up my butt *and* having to pay ridiculous amounts of money for it. My American neighbours are not so lucky.

A while ago, I underwent a bunch of testing due to my unexplained pelvic pain. As the GP couldn't figure out what was going on, she referred me to a gynecologist. However, she wanted to test me for STIs first, even though it was *very* unlikely I had one. As in, impossible because I'd never had sex. She wanted to rule them out for the gynecologist, who would want to see that the testing had been done and could move on to looking for other issues. It would simplify the process. I shrugged and said okay, not interested in fighting about it if it would make things easier with the specialist. Of course, the tests came back negative.

I didn't think much of this experience until a friend mentioned she'd had the exact same thing happen to her. As a virgin, she had been forced to go through an STI test for vaginal pain. Her story was the same as mine, except for one key difference. She was an American, so she had had to pay out of pocket for that unnecessary test.

Credit card debt is often the answer for those with chronic illnesses. Some wrack up thousands of dollars of debt in pursuit of a solution to their health problems. Tests and medications cost money, and it's frustrating because those tests often come back negative and those medications are often useless. But you need to try them in order to get to the next step in the treatment process. Even in Canada, health care bills can pile up if you don't have insurance.

For those who are sick and can't afford health care, it just sucks. When I see people rising up to help others who are going through financial difficulties, whether it's random people sending PayPal gifts to a friend on Facebook who admits she's struggling or dropping by with a load of groceries, it gives me hope.

When friends assure me they wouldn't let me starve if I ran out of money, it gives me a measure of safety. When my doctor tells me we'll keep trying until we find something that works, I nod tiredly, but I'm glad someone else isn't giving up.

When you're sick and struggling, you find community to survive. You find support. You find help. Even healthy people can't really do life alone, so it's foolish to think that you can. You can't always give back to that community, but you can thank them. You can show appreciation to the friends and family who stick with you, who value you, who are understanding when you are depressed, angry, annoyed, sick, or anxious. And when you're able, you give your time, understanding, and friendship in return.

I am extraordinarily fortunate to have multiple friends and support systems, but it took me a long time to accept those systems. Many with chronic illnesses are too exhausted to go looking, too anxious from past hurts to reach out. That loneliness bears down on anxiety like a kraken crushing a sloop at sea. That anxiety increases tenfold when there's no one to lean on.

Sometimes all you can manage is one step in the direction of community—whether that step is joining an online support group, reaching out to an old friend, or calling a family member. It might not feel like much, but that small movement may be worth it, even if it takes Amanda Brotzman levels of determination. It may also hurt. But you want the people around you to be like your anxiety—guaranteed to come back.

11

IF ONLY I HAD MORE FAITH

"That your daughter's gift causes her to invite pain into herself, and project pain into others, suggests something about what's going on inside her.... A cursory assessment says that on some level, she feels she deserves it. And she feels others deserve it as well."[1]

— DR. FADLAN, *CARVE THE MARK* BY
VERONICA ROTH

"*I* often feel that people (maybe especially the church) think I'm not trying hard enough," says Allison, a part-time bank teller with chronic fatigue syndrome/myalgic encephalomyelitis. "If I only exercised more, or drank more coffee, or took the right vitamins, or went to the right chiropractor, then I wouldn't be so tired all the time! Or if I had more faith, then God could heal me! These ideas are so hard to combat. They tie heavy burdens of responsibility for things we have no control

152 | ALLISON ALEXANDER

over and that are the loving and severe mercies of a sovereign God, and place them on our backs instead."

As Allison notes, religion can bring another level of complexity to chronic illness.[2] I grew up in a conservative Christian environment, and I've noticed that, as a group, Christians have a reputation for being judgmental. This is why I'm sometimes embarrassed to describe myself as a Christian, even though I continue to have faith as an adult (though it has significantly changed from what it was when I was a child).

The very humility Christ displayed, a trait we are supposed to model, sometimes gets shunted aside in favour of considering ourselves "chosen ones" or divinely directed to tell others how to turn away from their sin. There is a movement in Christianity called prosperity theology (or "health and wealth" gospel) that is especially damaging to poor and suffering people, because it suggests if we're not happy, healthy, and wealthy, we must not have enough faith. If we just prayed more, or read our Bible more, or went to church, we'd be as content as Groot, as healthy as Captain America, and as rich as Tony Stark.

Kate Bowler, a divinity professor with cancer, tackles this topic in her book *Everything Happens for a Reason: And Other Lies I've Loved*.

"'Everything happens for a reason.' The only thing worse than saying that is pretending that you know the reason. I've had hundreds of people tell me the reason for my cancer. Because of my sin. Because of my unfaithfulness. Because God is fair. Because God is unfair. Because of my aversion to Brussels sprouts. I mean, no one is short of reasons. So if people tell you this, make sure you are there when they go through the cruelest moments of their lives, and start offering your own. When someone is drowning, the only thing worse than failing to throw them a life preserver is handing them a reason."[3]

People are problem-solvers. They want to know *why* so that they can fix it. And fixing problems is easiest when they're not your own.

The other day, a friend sent a string of text messages out of the blue, saying she'd had the *exact* same health problems I was experiencing, but she'd found the spiritual root of her unhealthiness and was now free of her symptoms. She was praying for healing and freedom like that for me, that I would find the root of whatever sin was causing my sickness. She texted me again the next day to see if her prayers had cured me.

They hadn't. Because God hadn't pointed a finger at me to say, "You are cursed with pain until you, or people around you, pray harder to make up for when you ran that red light last week!" That's not a God I want to believe in.

I know from experience that mental health and physical health are deeply connected (one can cause the other to spiral, and vice versa), so if this woman found some spiritual peace that impacted her health in a positive way, that's wonderful. But every body is different, and God doesn't take pain away simply because we pray hard enough.

But many believe God does exactly that. Some Christians suggest that if you're sick, or depressed, or overwhelmed, you must not be trusting God enough. Either that, or you must deserve what you're going through. They sound like the friends of Job in the Bible, who tell the poor, suffering man that he must have done something to displease God (Job 8–22). They tell him to pray more, to ask for forgiveness, and to determine what he's done wrong so he can be healed. However, the Bible describes Job as a righteous man who does nothing to earn the terrible things that happen to him.

Suggesting it's my fault that I'm sick, that I just need more faith or more prayers said over me, is a misunderstanding of God's purpose for the world. And it's an incredibly damaging attitude to encounter, because I'm tempted to believe it when I'm at my weakest.

The thought of *what did I do to deserve this?* comes so naturally to me when I'm in pain. I feel the need for justice in the world and in my life. So I view my suffering through a lens of punishment and rail at God because I don't deserve it—but secretly, I'm afraid that I do.

JUDGING IS EASY, LOVING IS HARD

In the novel *Carve the Mark* by Veronica Roth, characters have supernatural abilities called currentgifts. Cyra Noavek's currentgift is not quite like the others; she can't see into the future or swap memories with someone or manipulate other people's emotions. Instead, her currentgift is chronic pain, which flits across her skin in the form of currentshadows every day, all day, and consumes her life. She can project this pain onto others, so her brother uses her as a weapon against his enemies. Cyra lives in a brutal warrior society, where her people carve the marks of their kills on their arms and murder each other for sport. And because people suspect currentgifts evolve from the essence of your being, Cyra's doctor suggests that, deep down, Cyra thinks she deserves, and others deserve, to be in pain.

Cyra feels like she's broken, just like I do. Sometimes I think I'm only a mere shadow of what a human should be. Unfixable. Unlovable.

It's only after Cyra meets and becomes friends with Akos, someone who truly cares about her, that she wonders if she has it wrong. There comes a time in the story when she is forced to torture him, but she is able to pull back her gift from harming him, a feat she's never managed to do before.

"On some level, I felt like I, and everyone else, deserved pain," she narrates. "One thing I knew, deep in my bones, was that Akos Kereseth did not deserve it."[4]

It is through receiving and pouring out unconditional love that Cyra comes to understand the world isn't as black and white as she'd like it to be. By the end of the series, Cyra doesn't believe she has the right to assume who deserves pain and who doesn't.

Though my focus is largely on Christianity in this chapter, as I have had some intense (both positive and negative) experiences in that quarter, judgemental attitudes can come from all kinds of sources. When you don't take someone's advice, they may think you're not trying hard enough and, therefore, it's your fault that you're sick. Some people believe in bad karma, generational sins that are passed on by your ancestors, or that the universe naturally punishes people to keep the world in balance. You might blame yourself for your illness because you ate the wrong food, smoked too much, or were at the wrong place at the wrong time. Or perhaps you just feel generally guilty about it, but aren't sure why.

Though some people continue to take it upon themselves to dole out judgment on others or on themselves, they're missing a crucial part about being human—the part where we choose humility over pride and love over judgment.

It is through believing I am loved—by God and by the people in my life—that I am able to value myself, too, and realize that pain isn't some quid pro quo system that God or anyone else has set up in order to punish me for misbehaviour.

In acknowledging this love, and feeling love for others, I am better able to accept my brokenness and accept the humanity of others around me in turn.

WHY, THOUGH?

Why, God? I thought as I dragged myself from the bathroom back to the seat next to my husband in the ER. I would make that trip, back and forth, every fifteen minutes for the next ten hours. Ten hours waiting all night in intense pain, and all I needed was a couple minutes of a doctor's time—a couple minutes to look at my chart, see that I had a urinary tract infection, and prescribe me an antibiotic.

But there was no way for me to rush the hospital's system. So I continued to pee blood, which felt more like acid, and sit on the dirty floor with my head in my husband's lap, because that was the least uncomfortable position I could find. When people afterward heard I had a UTI, the common response was, "I'm glad it wasn't serious." I appreciate the well wishes, but it certainly *felt* serious, as anyone who has experienced a bad UTI can attest.

I continue to ask that question, "Why me?" as similar symptoms persist even after the UTI has gone from my system, as weeks go by with no relief, and I have to deal with pelvic pain in addition to IBS. Doctors tested me for all the normal culprits—yeast infections, bacterial vaginosis, STIs, even ovarian cysts—with negative results. I'm stuck in this undiagnosed zone. Again.

Why, God? Why?

Why does pain exist? What is the point? It seems like a pretty stupid mechanism to me! Why would God make pain a part of being human *on purpose*?

"Much of the suffering on our planet has come about because of two principles that God built into creation: a physical world that runs according to consistent natural laws, and human freedom," writes Philip Yancey in *Where Is God When It Hurts?*[5]

Okay. I understand the principles that he is talking about here. Nature is a precise, complex system of natural laws that interconnect to make life possible, and pain does serve a useful purpose as part of those laws; it protects us. Put your hand too close to a flame and it hurts, signalling that we should pull away to avoid harming ourselves. A stomach ache may be caused by food poisoning and the body expelling the offending substances. The pain of a broken limb tells us we need medical attention.

There's another character in *Carve the Mark* who has a currentgift associated with pain, but it's the opposite of Cyra's. Vas's currentgift is the *inability* to feel pain, and he's a dangerous warrior because of it. It's only later in the novel that we get a little insight into his life: "Do you know I have to set alarms to eat and drink? And check myself constantly for broken bones and bruises," he says to Cyra. "It's exhausting, paying this much attention to your body."[6]

Patients with leprosy experience something similar—they may not even notice if they've been walking all day with a nail through their foot, if they've burned their hand by reaching into a fire, or if they've cut themselves. Their bodies can become damaged, ulcered, and diseased because they are numb to pain. Weirdly enough, pain is important to our health.

My problem, however, is when bodies go haywire, as mine has. I feel pain when I shouldn't. At some point, my body decided to add its own unique code to these laws, and the language it used was gibberish. It's not fair. Why would God allow it?

Reconciling the Creator of the universe with suffering is a larger topic that scholars wiser than I have struggled with and addressed in novel-length theses. But no matter how many Christian authors explain it away due to a free-willed universe or a consequence of sin, it's still difficult to wrap my mind around a loving God when intense pain is coursing through my body.

God is often compared to a caring parent, but if my mom and dad, who love me unconditionally, had the ability to stop my pain, they *absolutely would.* So why doesn't God?

"Modern objections to God are based on a sense of fair play and justice," writes Timothy Keller in *The Reason for God.* "People, we believe, *ought* not to suffer, be excluded, die of hunger or oppression. But the evolutionary mechanism of natural selection *depends* on death, destruction, and violence of the strong against the weak—these things are all perfectly natural."[7]

Keller touches on the feelings of injustice I experience when I'm in pain or see others in pain. Social justice, a movement that I support, is all about eliminating suffering—feeding the hungry, finding jobs for the poor, equalizing people groups, welcoming minorities, making peace, and asking forgiveness for the hurt we've caused. And yet, people still suffer everywhere and will continue to do so until the world is radically changed. I still do everything I can to halt suffering in my life and the lives of others, to find peace and joy, but if I decided that my life was *only* about avoiding suffering, there are some problems with that.

If my existence was all about avoiding suffering, then I might be okay with killing terminally ill patients, children born with disabilities, or others whose suffering affects their quality of life. But I'm not okay with those things. I believe those people deserve life, just as I do. There is a place for them in this world. There's a place for me in this world, even though my quality of life isn't perfect.

So if my purpose isn't happiness, pleasure, or avoiding suffering—what is it?

In the Bible, when a lawyer asks Jesus what the greatest commandment is, he replies that you should love God with all your heart and soul, and the second commandment is similar; love others as you love yourself (Matthew 22:37–39). This passage represents one of the biggest reasons I believe in God, because Jesus suggests my purpose is to be loved and to love in return. If that's the case, I can thrive in a world full of suffering, even if my body can't do what others can, even if I feel out of place and insufficient.

I still don't have the answer to *why* pain has to be part of this world. And I don't know if I ever will. Why couldn't we have robot bodies without pain receptors? Why couldn't we be intelligent amoebas without break-able bones? Why couldn't we all have Wolverine's regen-eration powers?

I only know that pain is part of what makes me human. I can question it all I want, but in the end, I just have to accept it. Faith is faith because we don't have all the answers.

"Sometimes intense suffering is part of this life for no reason at all," says Aaron, a Christian and musician who suffers from severe sciatica. "It happens. God allows it to happen. I don't like it, but I accept it.... Suffering helps us learn things and eventually overcome hardships to combat new ones. Because life is simply solving new problems once the old ones are defeated. There is no paradise until we get to heaven, because living a life of luxury, shelter, and safety will always eventually lead to entitled attitudes and a heart void of any gratitude."

CAN GOOD COME FROM SUFFERING?

"The way we experience God throwing the gauntlet to suffering is that suffering doesn't have the final word," says Jen Schlameuss-Perry, a Catholic pastoral associate and the author of *Comic Con Christianity*. "God built into it our ability to learn and grow from it, to become recon-ciled through it, and to offer it for the good of others.

"When the mystics and saints were sick, or persecuted,

or lonely, they kept their prayer life going and were able to see God's care for them in that suffering. They experienced revelations because it gave them time to put their hearts and their troubles into God's hands. They became perfectly reliant on God, and spent time in prayer that they otherwise wouldn't have had the time for, and were able to see clearly things they had never even thought to contemplate previously."

Jen says her suffering—the "rocks and mountains" that get in the way of life, which include watching her son face chronic illness—also reminds her of others who are in pain and spurs her to action on their behalf. When her kids are sick, their convenient access to health care reminds her of those in America who don't have that, or the women in Africa who sell everything they have to get medicine for their babies with malaria and might not even make it back in time to save them.

Nightcrawler, a character from the X-Men comics and TV series, says in an episode of the '90s animated series: "Our ability to understand God's purpose is limited, but we take comfort in the fact that his love is limitless."[8] His words are especially impactful because Nightcrawler knows suffering more than most; he is often shunned for his blue skin and demon-like appearance. Nightcrawler's deep devotion and gentle personality are rooted in his Catholic faith. Even though he says, "life will always be hard," he believes in a God who cares, and it impacts his outlook on life.

Like Jen and Nightcrawler, I believe good has come out of my suffering. For one thing, I suspect I'm more empathetic because of it, and this empathy impacts my life choices.

I have no idea where I would be now or what my personality would be like if I didn't struggle with a chronic illness. Would I care about other people? Would I be writing about the same topics I do now? Would I be married to the same person? Would I have different priorities? Maybe. I don't know. But I do know my pain has allowed me to see the world from a specific lens, and it's important for broken people to understand we are not alone. I can't go so far as to say I'm thankful for my pain and I certainly don't wish it on others, but I know good can come from it.

SUFFERING AS RESTORATION

I'm not alone in my suffering. However, I've learned not to dismiss my own pain by telling myself "someone else has it worse, so I should be thankful my pain isn't as bad." This is unhelpful because it just adds guilt to my already tumultuous emotions. Weighing my suffering against others' is a pointless exercise. Sure, someone else may have it "worse," but what does that even mean? What's the scale we're using for measuring suffering, and if mine weighs less than the next person's, does that mean I don't have a right to feel frustrated or sad? Can't we both suffer and both receive love and support?

I distinctly remember a friend telling me, when I admitted I was struggling with depression, "Yeah, but, your life's pretty good! You have a place to live, and friends, and a job. Try focusing on those things!"

She's right, I thought. *I should be feeling thankful, not sad and depressed. I'm a horrible person!*

I felt guilty for not being happy about the good things

in my life. After all, I could be a struggling orphan with no friends, no family, no health care. I could be a blind amputee, or a dying cancer patient. Their pain must be "worse" than mine, right?

There is a benefit to being thankful for the good things in my life. Gratitude has been scientifically proven to lower depression in chronic illness patients. "I'm struck that [the definition for gratitude] in no way precludes the presence of anger and sorrow," writes Katie Willard Virant in *Psychology Today*. "To be thankful for what one possesses does not mean that one cannot simultaneously feel grief for what one has lost."[9] These things are not mutually exclusive.

There's this really "fun" verse in the Bible that's super clear and not open to false, harmful interpretations *at all* (cue sarcastic tone):

"Whenever you face trials of any kind, consider it nothing but joy" (James 1:2, NRSV).

But, James, I can't just slap a smile on my face and pretend I'm not hurting—can I?

Turns out, I can. But it's not very healthy for my mind, body, or spirit. Pretending to be happy when you're really not is draining. I'm just lying to everyone around me, and the people who genuinely care about me don't actually want that, even if they sometimes say unhelpful things in an effort to cheer me up.

However, if you dig further into this verse and consider its context, you learn that the joy James refers to isn't a fake happiness. Our understanding of this passage is coloured by our culture's understanding of the word *joy*. When joy is viewed as a feeling, my ability to find joy in suffering is nonexistent. James, however, is already looking ahead to the world as it will be after God makes it perfect, and not as it is—something I'm not very good at because pain centres me in the here and now. But that kind of rejoicing is more of a choice, less of a feeling.

"The biblical view of things is resurrection—not a future that is just a *consolation* for the life we never had but a *restoration* of the life you always wanted," writes Timothy Keller in *The Reason for God.* "This means that every horrible thing that ever happened will not only be undone and repaired but will in some way make the eventual glory and joy even greater."

I like the idea of a future world where our suffering in this life is not just unravelled, but part of what makes the new world good. It's a restoration that builds on everything that has come before, instead of tearing down, using our brokenness for good instead of erasing it.

I can't believe in a God who tells me to just grin and bear my suffering, and I don't think the biblical writers did, either. Many of the Psalms, passages in the Bible that are usually lauded for their great praises and songs to God, are laments about pain and suffering. Those parts where the psalmist cries out to God in pain are there because it is human to do so, and God understands that.

In the end, pain and suffering in relation to my faith are still very much a mystery to me. I don't completely understand. I still wrestle with the question *why?*

"Ultimately, I have a God who chose to suffer with me," Jen says, "and Jesus' suffering was transformative for humanity; salvific and revelatory. I know that when I suffer, I don't suffer alone. I have a God who has suffered himself—who knows what I'm going through personally, cares about what I'm going through, and holds me through it. God doesn't allow my suffering to have the last word—God is the last word, and that word is love."

If you take nothing else from this chapter, take love. Take other people's love. Take God's. Take your own. And when you take in all that love, you might find yourself able to give it out to others, and that's pretty wonderful. Know that you have done nothing to "deserve" your pain. Try to set aside the judgment you feel from others and from yourself (easier said than done, I know). You don't need to meet any requirements to be loved.

THE MASS EFFECT OF RELIGION

"Amonkira, Lord of Hunters, grant that my hands be steady, my aim be true, and my feet swift. And should the worst come to pass, grant me forgiveness."[1]

— THANE KRIOS, *MASS EFFECT 2*

*I*n the video game *Mass Effect 2* by BioWare, a drell named Thane Krios joins Commander Shepard's crew. Just like the other characters aboard the *Normandy*, Thane is dedicated to stopping the Reapers from destroying the galaxy. He is also dying of a fictional illness called Kepral's syndrome. This disease plagues his species, causing their lungs to degrade because their bodies are not functional in the climates of most planets.

"Our lungs can't deal with the moisture," Thane explains. "Over time, the tissue loses its ability to absorb oxygen. It becomes harder to breathe. Eventually we suffocate."

Patrick Weekes, a member of the writing team for the

Mass Effect series, said that Kepral's syndrome was inspired by cystic fibrosis, a real-world illness that affects the digestive system and lungs.[2] However, Thane's illness isn't as harsh as cystic fibrosis because he was intended to be a functioning member of Shepard's team and needed to be able to move around doing missions (though, in *Mass Effect 3*, he is hospitalized because the illness has progressed too far).

While some might complain that you can't cure Thane in the futuristic Mass Effect universe, in which Shepard is literally brought back from the dead, I appreciate the inclusion of an incurable illness while I simultaneously weep at his inability to be part of my team in *Mass Effect 3*. Even with our understanding of science and medicine, incurable illnesses continue to exist and probably always will; BioWare embraces that reality by including disabled and sick characters in their games.

Thane also fascinates me because he is deeply religious, embracing a polytheistic faith. He refers to three deities throughout the games: Amonkira, Lord of Hunters; Arashu, Goddess of Motherhood and Protection; and Kalahira, Goddess of Oceans and the Afterlife. Since these gods represent very specific areas of life, it seems likely that there are more drell gods he simply doesn't mention. What's truly interesting about Thane is that he is an assassin, but he has a deep respect for life. He kills to create a better world and protect the innocent, but he knows the act of killing is still evil and prays for forgiveness. (Note: I said *interesting*, not *moral* or that I agree with these particular philosophies.)

"Prayers for the wicked must never be forsaken," Thane says upon his first appearance in *Mass Effect 2* as he

stands, head bowed, over the body of Nissana, a mercenary he just killed:

"Nissana and her men deserve what they got," Shepard
replies.

"Not for her. For me."

This acknowledgement of wrong seems contradictory
to some of his other statements, like this one: "An assassin
is a weapon. A weapon doesn't choose to kill. The one
who wields it does." This philosophy links to Thane's religion, for drell believe the soul and body are separate;
therefore, if his body is ordered to do something under a
contract, Thane is not responsible. He doesn't feel guilty
for killing, referring to his time as a contract assassin as
being "asleep for a long time," even though, because of
drells' eidetic memories, he can remember every last kill.
He maintains his soul knows right from wrong, but his
body doesn't.

"Drell minds are different from humans'," he says. "We
see our body as a vessel, and accept that it is not always
under our control."

I may not agree with all of Thane's philosophies
concerning responsibility, but I appreciate the way he
accepts his illness and tries to leave the world a better
place before he dies. A lot of my frustrations with illness
come from my desire to control my body. But if I
consider my body the same way Thane does his—as a
vessel that I can't always control—I can let go of some of
my frustration and move closer to acceptance.

Of course, it's difficult for me to let go of control—
even the illusion of it. A deep-seated need for control
seems to be part of human nature, because control gives
us a sense of security and understanding of how things

work. We even like the illusion of control—changing our appearances after a breakup to symbolize the change we hope to see inside ourselves, or shaving our heads because the hair's going to fall out from cancer treatment anyway. These small choices give us the illusion of power over a situation, and that mirage is comforting.

I "take control" of my illness by trying new medications, diets, exercises, treatments, and anything I can think of that might ease my pain.

Sometimes these things help, sometimes they make things worse, and sometimes they do nothing at all. They're definitely worth trying, because there's always the chance that they'll help, even if for a short time. But when the pain hits, and I'm frustrated that nothing I do seems to make it go away, the tension in my body increases along with my stress, which makes the pain worse.

The best thing I can do for my body in those moments is let go of my raging desire for control and accept that pain is happening and there's nothing I can do about it.

THE BENEFITS OF RELIGION AND SPIRITUALITY

Religion can either be a road to acceptance or an added stressor where chronic illness is concerned, depending on whether you are able to reconcile the existence of a deity with your suffering. Perhaps that is why studies have shown mixed results in finding whether religion and spirituality are related to higher pain levels, lower pain levels, or unrelated to pain severity.

"Hindu traditions promote coping with suffering by accepting it as a just consequence and understanding that suffering is not random," writes Sarah M. Whitman in *The Journal of Pain* article "Pain and Suffering as Viewed by the Hindu Religion."[3]

Hindus may find comfort in believing their suffering has a purpose and that it does not affect their soul, attempting to gain a level of detachment from their pain:

"But while the body may be in pain, the Self or soul is not affected or harmed," Whitman writes. "Patients may gain comfort by viewing the pain as only a temporary condition and one that does not affect their inner Self."[4]

Sarah—a mom, English teacher, and Muslim—says, "It is said that no illness or injury touches a human being without God's permission. We are here on earth for a time, and our time here is a test. He has provided us with countless blessings to help make life here bearable, but He said, too, that we will be tested."

Sarah says much of what she's learned about faith and illness came from watching her mother endure cancer for years before passing away in 2008:

"Yes, she had moments of despair and anguish," Sarah says, "but I also know that she had a steadfast faith in God and that her suffering was for a purpose... perhaps to expiate her sins in life? Perhaps to serve as a lesson to others? Who knows. But she truly believed it was to bring her closer to God. To serve as an example of His infinite love and wisdom.

"The doctors often marvelled at how healthy she looked, and commented throughout her years of illness how they couldn't understand what was allowing her to pull through each time they called us to tell us she probably

wouldn't make it through the night. But she knew. It was
her faith."

Sarah mentioned that everything we're given in life—
the good and bad—is a reminder of its temporariness. The
Quran frequently refers to death befalling everybody; no
one can escape it.

While sometimes the reality of death is scary, at other
times it's a relief because I want to escape my pain. Faith
is a comfort because I want to believe there is a pain-free
existence waiting for me, though that doesn't stop me
from trying to find relief in this world.

FAITH AND MEDICINE

"Muslims believe that there is no illness that does not also
have a cure," Sarah says. "That belief is what inspired the
Muslims of history to pursue medical knowledge. So faith
and practical application (i.e., medicines and treatments)
go hand in hand.

"There may be a minority view that you should just
put your faith in God for a cure, but it is just that: a very
small minority. We have always believed that *because* of
your faith you should seek to do all you can. God helps
those who help themselves."

Some religious people question whether they are truly
being "faithful" by seeking medical attention. They
emphasize the spiritual over the physical, believing that
true faith means waiting for God to do everything. Thus,
they spend their time praying instead of doing.

I wish I could just pray away my illness, but it hasn't
worked so far, and I don't think God discourages people

from seeking relief from their pain through science. I wonder if God gets tired of people asking fir her to do every little thing for them—things that they could accomplish on their own. "Heal my infection so I don't have to go to the doctor to get antibiotics, God." "Watch over my niece so I don't have to pay attention to her, God." "Tie my shoelaces, God." God is not an excuse to be lazy, and it's inaccurate to equate faithfulness with relying on God for everything.

Regardless of God's attitude toward us, there are scientific studies that suggest religion and spirituality are valuable tools for coping with chronic illness. Prayer can serve as a positive distraction during illness, thinking about God can help relieve anxiety, and believing in a higher power can contribute to positive mental coping.[5] The social support from religious communities is also valuable in coping with illness.

Many religions, including Christianity, Islam, Hinduism, and Buddhism, encourage believers to focus on healthy emotions, like peace, joy, and love. When not twisted by fundamentalists, spirituality encourages people to treat others well, too. Grace and forgiveness are at the heart of Christianity, and peace and commitment at the centre of Islam; Hinduism reinforces right conduct, and Buddhism is about harmony and peace from suffering.

"My faith also commands that we see everyone around us as worthy of love and compassion. That's non-negotiable," says Sarah.

Altruism itself is, in fact, healthy for us. It can release endorphins, give us satisfaction, and help distract us from our problems.[6] This implies that being committed to a religion that encourages we love one another is also good for our minds and bodies. Too bad altruism isn't a cure for illness itself, or the world would be overflowing with do-gooders.

SUFFERING AND SELFLESSNESS

Thane's final act in *Mass Effect 3* is one of self-sacrifice to save others. As he lays dying in the hospital due to loss of blood and his illness, he says a prayer that his son, Kolyat (and Shepard, if the player chooses to participate), finishes for him:

> Kalahira, mistress of inscrutable deaths, I
>   ask forgiveness.
> Kalahira, whose waves wear down stone
>   and sand—
> Kalahira, wash the sins from this one and
>   set him on the distant shore of the
>   infinite spirit.
> Kalahira, this one's heart is pure, but
>   beset by wickedness and contention.
> Guide this one to where the traveler never
>   tires, the lover never leaves, the
>   hungry never starve.
> Guide this one, Kalahira, and she will be
>   a companion to you as she was
>   to me.[7]

A cutscene with a full prayer is uncommon in a video game, and it is a testament to how Thane's faith is such a large part of his character.

If you are playing female Shepard, she asks Kolyat why

the last verse says "she," and he replies that Thane's final prayer is for her, not for himself. He is asking his gods to watch over Shepard. Even during his dying breaths, Thane is at peace and is more concerned about another.

Thane reminds me that illness isn't an excuse to be selfish. It's easy to get wrapped up in my own pain, to focus on nothing else but feeling better, and to expect everyone around me to attend to my needs. But focusing solely on myself results in bitterness, anger, and lots of horrible emotions that I have no desire to experience. I'd much rather be at peace with myself and my illness and be available to empathize with others.

My relationship with a God who suffers with me has been a source of peace. It's also a solace for many others in similar situations. Just as Thane finds peace with his gods, Christians, Buddhists, Hindus, Muslims, and people of other faiths have found meaning in spiritual practices that encourage them to reconcile the nature of suffering with how the world works.

Faith can make a path for us to be selfless, to respect others and ourselves, and to make peace with our illnesses. I believe this to be true and hope spirituality will continue to be respected throughout the world as a means of coping in difficult times and as a way of life that gives purpose to those who choose it.

13

TO HAVE IT OVER WITH

"When he was burying me, Rhyme, I couldn't move. Not an inch. For an instant I was desperate to die. Not to live, just to have it over with. I understood how you feel."[1]

— AMELIA SACHS, *THE BONE COLLECTOR* BY
JEFFERY DEAVER

*Y*ou can tell me how "life is meaningful" while I'm sitting on the toilet with pain squishing my gut, and it won't mean anything to me. Intellectually, the words may register, but it's difficult to want to live when you are suffering, depressed or not.

The Bone Collector, a crime thriller novel-turned-movie by Jeffrey Deaver, features a brilliant criminologist and quadriplegic. Due to an accident at a crime scene that crushed his vertebrae, he can only move his head and his left ring finger.

Lincoln Rhyme is the opposite of the "inspirational"

type of disabled character. Instead, he's sarcastic, lonely, and bitter.

He is also determined to commit doctor-assisted suicide. At the beginning of the story, he meets with Dr. William Berger, a representative of a pro-euthanasia group, to convince the doctor to do the deed. Rhyme has gone through skull traction, ventilators, nerve stimulators, catheters, surgery, ulcers, hypotension, bedsores, and phantom pain, among other things. But he doesn't even bother going over those stressors with the doctor, instead simply telling him about the latest "wrinkle" in his life: autonomic dysreflexia.

> "The problem had been occurring more often recently. Pounding heartbeat, off-the-charts blood pressure, raging headaches. It could be brought on by something as simple as constipation. He explained that nothing could be done to prevent it except avoiding stress and physical constriction."[2]

Rhyme has lost everything due to his condition—even his wife, whom he promptly divorced once he realized she was only staying with him out of pity. He can't visit crime scenes anymore. He can't even leave his bed, much less his home. He feels useless, he's in constant discomfort and pain, and he just wants it to end. Who can blame him? His life sounds miserable.

CHRONIC ILLNESS AND SUICIDAL THOUGHTS

For the chronically ill, the desire to end things may or may not be accompanied by clinical depression. Depression can cause suicidal thoughts, but so can being in pain 24/7. Depression can be triggered by something else and then be exacerbated by the illness, or the illness can trigger the depression. The two often come as a package deal because bodies and minds are interconnected, but it's important to distinguish that depression related to chronic illness or pain is not necessarily illogical. Being in pain all the time... I don't know how to describe it, how to *really* describe it, to someone who's never experienced it before. But I can say there's nothing twisted about a desire to be done with that suffering.

For Holly, a thirty-one-year-old with undifferentiated connective tissue disease, fibromyalgia, avoidant restrictive food intake disorder, and anxiety, her depression was triggered by the loss of the most important friendship in her life.

"As the well of grief opened up, it was like peeling back an onion of unhealth," she recalls.

The stress she experienced caused her physical pain to skyrocket and revealed a tendency for codependency and an addiction to meeting others' needs. She felt like her life had lost its purpose, and her illness compounded the stress, plunging her into a time of darkness.

"I spent hours upon hours hiding in my closet hoping I would never have to come back out," Holly says. "When your brain is so confused, when your body is in unrelenting pain from head to toe, it feels unbearable to keep going, the world feels terrifying. Your depression becomes so thick that you cannot see anything besides the terrifying. You can't see beauty, you can't see hope, you can't see redemption. And when you can only see the horrific around you, when your brain feels horrific and your body feels horrific, you want out."

It took therapy, the right medication combo, and lots of time for Holly to stabilize and experience suicidal thoughts less frequently. "My life stopped," she says. "I took a medical leave of absence from work, slept ten to twelve hours a night, went to therapy four hours a week, read books while I sobbed, learned slowly to take care of myself, to spend money on myself, time on myself. I backed out of almost all commitments and many relationships. I stayed at home almost always, changed my phone number and disappointed many people as I set tons of boundaries. And it is important to note that all of that required TONS of privilege that many people do not have."

Holly's experience was difficult enough, but those who don't have as much privilege may take longer to address mental health issues. Or, the horrifying reality is, without the proper support, they may end up dead. Chronic illness does not offer a way out; it is a painful existence. Living with it requires the love, community, and support of other people.

YOU CAN'T LOGIC AWAY THE SUICIDE

In *The Bone Collector*, Lincoln Rhyme gets drawn into a homicide case and postpones his plans to commit suicide so he can help solve the mystery. A police officer, Amelia Sachs, becomes his eyes and ears on the scene, and they end up falling in love with each other.

Throughout the story, Sachs tries to convince Rhyme to choose life after the case is over. Her first argument is that avoiding pain is "cowardly," to which he responds, "if that's true then why anesthetize patients before surgery? Why sell aspirin? Why fix broken arms? Why is Prozac the most prescribed medicine in America? Sorry, but there's nothing intrinsically good about pain."

She then says that he can contribute so much to the community with his knowledge of forensics and experience as a detective, to which he replies, "But who says we should contribute anything to life? Besides, the corollary is I might contribute something bad. I might cause some harm too. To myself or someone else."

She then switches tactics, arguing that life is full of challenges and maybe a cure will be discovered, but he has a response for every point she makes.

> "'Sachs, I'm tired,' he said earnestly. 'I can't tell you how tired I am. You know how hard life is to start with. Pile on a whole mountainful of… burdens. Washing, eating, crapping, making phone calls, buttoning shirts, scratching your nose… Then pile on a thousand more. And more after that.'"

Rhyme doesn't have brain fog like Holly did during her depression. He's not mentally incapacitated. He understands the consequences of his decision. He's just exhausted and wants life to be over.

Sachs doesn't understand, refusing to accept his decision. She only gets an inkling of Rhyme's experience when she is almost buried alive during the case. "For an instant I was desperate to die," she tells him. It is, perhaps, this experience that causes her to stop arguing with Rhyme. She accepts his decision, though she doesn't agree with it. "All I can say is, I just don't want you to do it," she finally says.

This statement is, perhaps, the most impactful one she could have made. Knowing that someone cares about you is a powerful thing, though that in itself is not necessarily enough to prevent someone's suicide.

SUICIDAL THOUGHTS AS A CONDITION

Some do not arrive at their decision to end their lives as logically as Rhyme does. Many suicidal people say, even in the midst of depression, that they do not *want* to take their own lives. If we consider suicide as something that happens *to* people, like a car crash or cancer, instead of something they *commit*, we may understand their perspective better.

"You get to a place of complete and utter numbness, where you feel like you don't exist, like you're a bizarre holograph," says Sharon Blady, mental health advocate and previous minister of health for the province of Manitoba.

> "You wonder why anyone would miss you, because you don't feel like you're really there. That emptiness, that lack of feeling, that numbness is overwhelming and debilitating. Any sense of agency you have in that situation is qualified in that you literally feel like you have no other option. Anything else you try or think you can try is not going to stop the extreme pain or the extreme numbness."

Sharon, who has struggled with depression, suicidal

thoughts, and cancer, often gets triggered by anxiety. After experiencing two major episodes of suicidal thoughts over the years, she says that "it's like someone has taken over a remote control of my brain. They're flipping through the channels in a different way, frequency, and volume. You get sucked in to believing [suicidal thoughts that you're worthless] because on some level it is you, but it's a toxic version of you... I wouldn't call [suicide] true agency because of the way that thing is controlling the remote."

If we consider suicidal thoughts as a condition, then they require treatment just like any other illness. Therapy, medication, and proper support may contribute to a healthier mental state.

"What happened to me was this idea of reframing," Sharon says. "When my youngest one was diagnosed with anxiety and ADD and thought that he was broken, I said to him, 'You're not broken; you're like an X-Man. You have mutant superpowers.'

"If you can get through the dark, shitty parts of depression, you come out with some pretty amazing skill sets on the other side. Grounded realism, empathy, compassion... I wouldn't wish my mental health profile on anyone and at the same time I can't imagine having accomplished certain things otherwise. It's about managing it, harnessing it. It's about figuring out triggers and distracting or keeping that part of the brain preoccupied. When you learn to manage these things, you learn to put things in perspective."

Sharon says when people tried to talk to her about her

mental health, she didn't feel valued, she didn't feel heard, she didn't feel listened to. She appreciated when people spent more time listening than talking, letting her express herself and demonstrating that her feelings were valid. What she needed was acceptance and non-judgment. "Accept that this is how I see the world right now in this moment and that it is overwhelming right now," she says.

WARNING SIGNS

For people with chronic illnesses, suicide may not always present itself in the same way as with physically healthy people. Suicidal thoughts in physically healthy people may look like having mood swings, increasing use of alcohol or drugs, developing personality disorders, feeling hopeless, and doing self-destructive things. Suicidal thoughts for those with chronic illnesses may include those symptoms as well, but are often specifically linked to loneliness and feeling like a burden and an outcast.[3] That, along with the excruciating pain and discomfort, may bring us to question the point of our existence.

Warning signs of suicidal thoughts may include:

- Feeling like the people in your life would be better off without you.
- Talking less because you feel like your opinion is unimportant.
- Feeling empty.
- Feeling extreme loneliness.
- Avoiding everyone.
- Feeling like your thoughts and anxiety are out of control.

- Being angry at yourself for your own pain.
- Believing you don't belong in the world.
- Feeling like things, animals, or people you love don't bring you joy anymore.
- Staring blankly into space for hours.
- Purposefully avoiding medication or pain relievers when you need them.

It's useful to recognize your own warning signs, because if you know what's happening, you might be able to do something about it. I can tell when I'm about to spiral into depression because I suddenly feel lost about what to do with my free time. Nothing I normally like doing sounds fun. I'll find myself on the couch, staring out the window, and then realize, "Oh, I'm depressed. That's what's happening." Then, I'll ask myself whether I missed taking my antidepressant the day before; I'll tell someone how I'm feeling so they can encourage me and I'm reminded others care; I'll go for a walk or sit outside; or, sometimes, I'll just put on a TV show, let myself feel depressed, and wait for a new day.

Giving yourself space to feel how you feel can potentially eliminate feelings of anxiety or illness. However, if you find yourself thinking about concrete ways to kill yourself, it's time to get someone else involved and to take steps to decide that your life is worth continuing.

EMBRACING LIFE

At the end of *The Bone Collector*, Amelia Sachs sits with Lincoln Rhyme as he puts a glass of brandy to his lips, which contains dissolved pills that will end his life. Sachs doesn't agree with his decision, but she's accepted it. She has decided being there for him is more important than letting him do this alone. But then, they're interrupted.

Detective Lon Sellitto, Rhyme's ex-partner, unexpectedly drops by to inform them that a bomb went off at the United Nations an hour before and links the perp to the case Rhyme just solved. Rhyme is fascinated by the juicy details of the case but says he can't help them. Except, as Sellitto continues to describe the case, Rhyme gets drawn in. The fact that a little girl's life is in danger cements his decision.

He agrees to work the case, and Sachs dumps his tainted brandy out the window with a smile, marking the conclusion of this novel and the beginning of a detective series featuring the two of them.

The abruptness in Rhyme's change of heart works in a novel because it gives the ending a little bit of humour intermingled with hope. I can't say whether a similar situation would turn so quickly in real life, but it's important to note that several things impacted Rhyme's decision.

Rhyme narrates earlier that Amelia Sachs' romantic feelings for him are one of the reasons he decides to commit suicide—because he can't see a future for them. But at the end, it's also one of the biggest reasons he chooses to live. Knowing someone cares about you is a big deal. You can look at relationships, romantic or platonic, as opportunities to be disappointed and hurt, or you can look at them with hope—that perhaps this person will continue to care about you just the way you are.

Rhyme also finds hope through passion and purpose. He loves solving puzzles and doing detective work. He can still do those things, though the job looks much more different than it used to because he can't physically be in the field. Sickness often means learning to do things differently than healthy people. It may mean finding completely new things to be passionate about or to preoccupy ourselves with. It may mean feeling useless, but accepting that we are valuable for our ability to love.

When my passion for the things I love is drained away by the throes of depression and I feel like my life has no meaning, I still remember what it felt like to be hopeful, and I want that feeling back. There are many times when I can't argue for my existence, when I can't logic away feelings of worthlessness, but I hear all the people who care about me saying, "You matter." Even if it's only one voice saying it, it makes a difference.

I can't argue away my desire to end the pain, but I can find hope if I'm willing to look for it. And if I'm too tired to begin the search today, I can rest and wait for tomorrow.

In the end, embracing life is not about expecting health and happiness. Life is painful, quite literally for those of us with chronic conditions. It's stressful. It's difficult. But it matters. We matter. If I stop believing that, I stop living, and I choose to embrace life even when it hurts.

14

SUPERHEROES ARE SICK

"I wish it need not have happened in my time."[1]

— FRODO BAGGINS, *THE FELLOWSHIP OF THE RING*

Though much of pop culture tells me sick people aren't valuable, Samwise Gamgee says, "There is some good in this world, Mr. Frodo." I've managed to find some positive representations in these chapters, and I hope to discover more in the future.

As it turns out, and despite what culture says or doesn't say, superheroes *are* sick. We don't have to feel mighty to be worthy.

We may never "win" our fight, but it's not about winning. We may be considered "invalid" by some, but we're invaluable. We may be exhausted, but we don't have to push ourselves to "go beyond" in order to prove something. We may feel unworthy, but we are loved. We may want the pain to end, but even scraps of hope can make life worth sticking around for.

Pain sucks. Chronic illness sucks. It's not fair.

Like Frodo, who gets stuck lugging around a toxic ring that exerts its will over him, I wish sickness hadn't happened to me. Gandalf has something wise to say in response:

"So do all who live to see such times. But that is not for them to decide. All we have to decide is what to do with the time that is given us."

Moving toward peace through pain begins with accepting that pain exists in the first place, as much as I'd like to avoid it, and then deciding that I want to live anyway. For me, that acceptance is a process, and it doesn't mean giving up hope.

THREE TYPES OF SUFFERING

The Buddhist tradition defines three types of suffering that are useful to contemplate:

1) Physical and mental pain (such as what you feel after breaking a leg or when a friend dies);

2) the changing nature of life, and how we are hyperaware that a pleasant experience will come to an end; and

3) anxiety.

Going through the first type of suffering, physical and

mental pain, is unavoidable, but acceptance allows me to co-exist with it and confront the next two types.

I'm glad someone put the second type of suffering into words, because I experience this phenomenon during many of the days, hours, or minutes when I am pain-free or having a particularly joyful moment. Because I experience pain and sickness so often, I'm conscious that the good moment will not last. Then sad, unwanted feelings intrude into my happy-land like the Ring poisoning Gollum's mind.

I am also intimately familiar with the third type of suffering. It's when I go beyond the suffering of the moment, anxious about what might happen or what happened in the past and what I should or should not have done about it. I struggle with anxiety and over-thinking things. This type of suffering is dumping tons of unnecessary thoughts on top of "this hurts and I want it to stop." For me, that thought pattern often goes something like this:

It's not fair that this hurts so much. Look how much I'm suffering compared to all the healthy people in the world; woe is me. Although, I'm not going hungry in a third-world country. I have health care. I'm not homeless. I'm not being tortured. Torture might be worse than this. I'm not dying. I shouldn't be feeling grief at all from this, because those people have it so much worse than I do. Well... now I feel guilty. But ow, this hurts so much. What if it never stops hurting? What if I have to call my husband away from work to take me to the hospital? What if...? But maybe...? How will I...?

Buddhists would suggest practicing mindfulness to alleviate these anxieties, noting the differences between the pain itself and my experience of it. I find this a useful concept to practice, because "letting go," to me, means accepting things as they are (being sick) instead of trying to make them into something they are not (being cured). I can work on accepting that I am sick and strive to find peace through my sickness without basing that peace on being healed.

There's something else I like to take from the Buddhist handbook: practicing loving-kindness and compassion. This is also apparent in other religions and people with no religion or spirituality, of course, but Buddhists make special note of it as something to consistently practice.

I find that compassion, toward myself and others, helps clear my mind of the frustration, guilt, and impatience that come from wanting what I don't have. Compassion is like the broomstick that's clearing away the unwanted, dusty emotions that cling to the floor of my brain. And I have to keep sweeping regularly because the dust keeps collecting. But if I do, I find my well-being comes from somewhere other than my wants and desires. I've found purpose in life through faith in a God who loves me and through relationships with others.

You may find meaning in other core values, such as altruism, treating others with compassion; developing positive characteristics like patience, generosity, and gratitude; and growing as a person. Developing these values can give us purpose, a purpose that helps us find meaning in life.

THE VALUE OF ACCEPTANCE

Science backs the value of acceptance. A *PubMed* study found that "Greater acceptance of pain was associated with reports of lower pain intensity, less pain-related anxiety and avoidance, less depression, less physical and psychosocial disability, more daily uptime, and better work status in persons seeking treatment for chronic pain."[2]

Accepting suffering doesn't mean I can't still address the malfunctions of my body or should stop taking care of it. It also doesn't mean I can't have desires and goals, or can't want to be well; it's when my joy is dependent on receiving my desires that there's a problem. If all the positive emotions of joy, peace, satisfaction, happiness, and hope are tied up in getting better, I would probably be a very sad, angry, and frustrated person, since the word *chronic* isn't attached to my illness for fits and giggles. And while I am those things sometimes, those emotions don't define me.

In *The View from Rock Bottom*, author Stephanie Tait suggests refocusing our pain by thinking about ourselves less and others more. This doesn't mean simply ignoring our pain in an effort to distract ourselves by doing good deeds, but it takes into account the very nature of our suffering and how we might use it for good.

> "[This healing] is not someone trying to overcome depression by visiting terminal patients in order to guilt herself into more gratefulness; it is my friend who vulnerably published a memoir about her own mental health struggles in an effort to erase the stigmas and bring hope to others waging a similar war," Tait writes. "It is not the deeply toxic suggestion that victims should 'forgive and forget' horrific acts of abuse; it is my friend who bravely went public with her story of sexual abuse

by a former pastor and began passionately advocating for necessary change in churches all around the country."[3]

By turning our pain into a tool that we can use to help better the world around us, we are finding life in the ashes.

Instead of wishing my life looked different, I acknowledge my pain exists and that suffering is part of my life. I also remind myself that my pain is *not shameful*. This is still a concept I struggle with, because my illnesses involve topics that are socially inappropriate to talk about, like bowel movements and female genitalia. I feel embarrassed about it. I badly want my life to be different. Yet, if I practice being with my life just the way it is, if I use my superpowers of pain and illness for good, I can find peace.

In *The Lord of the Rings*, Frodo carries his burden step by step all the way to Mordor. He can't do it on his own, just like I can't survive my illness on my own. There are Sams willing to carry me up Mount Doom if I let them. Of course, I don't get to toss my illness into a boiling pit of lava, as much as I wish that were the case. I just get to keep trudging down a never-ending path. But sometimes I glimpse white shores ahead. I find pockets of rest in the midst of suffering. There may be no end in sight, but the end isn't why I'm continuing on.

As I take each step, I remind myself that I am valuable. I am worthwhile. I am loved. And that's what makes me super.

NOTES

FOREWORD

1. "I'm not your inspiration, thank you very much | Stella Young." *YouTube*, uploaded by TED, 9 Jun. 2014, https://www.youtube.com/watch?v=8K9Gg164Bsw
2. Onyx, Fay. *Resources*. Writing Alchemy, 13 Jan. 2018, https://writingalchemy.net/resources/
3. *Crip Camp: A Disability Revolution*. Directed by Nicole Newnham and James Lebrecht. Netflix, 2020.
4. *Special*. Directed by Anna Dokoza. Netflix, 2019–2021.
5. Sjunneson Henry, Elsa, et al. *Disabled People Destroy Science Fiction*. Uncanny Magazine, 2018.
6. Sjunneson Henry, Elsa, et al. *Fate Accessibility Toolkit*. Evil Hat Productions, 2019.

1. SUPERHEROES AREN'T SICK

1. *Doctor Strange*. Dir. Scott Derrickson. Marvel Studios, 2016. Film.
2. Mayo Clinic Staff. "Irritable bowel syndrome." *Mayo Clinic*, https://www.mayoclinic.org/diseases-conditions/irritable-bowel-syndrome/symptoms-causes/syc-20360016

2. INVALID: A DIRTY WORD

1. Headley, Maria Dahvana. *Magonia*. New York: HarperCollins, 2015.
2. "Scott's Tots," *The Office*, S6, Ep12. NBC, December 3, 2009. Television.
3. "Pilot," *Speechless*, S1, Ep1. ABC, September 21, 2016. Television.
4. Praderio, Caroline. "LGBTQ patients reveal their exhausting, infuriating, and surprisingly common struggles at the doctor's office." *Insider*, May 31, 2019, https://www.insider.com/lgbtq-healthcare-doctors-health-disparities-2018-4

5. McDowell, Emily. "Empathy Cards for Serious Illness." *Emily McDowell & Friends*, May 3, 2015, https://emilymcdowell.com/blogs/all/105537926-empathy-cards-for-serious-illness

3. DOCTOR HOUSE KNOWS BEST. SOMETIMES. MAYBE.

1. "Holding On," *House*, S8 Ep21. NBC, May 14, 2012. Television.
2. Chainey, Naomi. "Comment: Where is Chronic Illness Represented in Popular Culture?" *The Feed*, October 6, 2016, https://www.sbs.com.au/news/the-feed/comment-where-is-chronic-illness-represented-in-popular-culture
3. "Pilot," *House*, S1, Ep1. NBC, November 16, 2004. Television.
4. Larsen, Pamela D. *Lubkin's Chronic Illness: Impact and Intervention*. Burlington: Jones & Bartlett Learning, 2014.
5. "The Softer Side," *House*, S5, Ep16. NBC, February 23, 2009. Television.
6. "Distractions," *House*, S2, Ep12. NBC, February 14, 2006. Television.

4. GIVE IT ONE MILLION PERCENT

1. "One for All," *My Hero Academia*, S3, Ep11. Adult Swim, June 16, 2018. Television.
2. Miserandino, Christine. "The Spoon Theory." *But You Don't Look Sick*, 2003, https://butyoudontlooksick.com/articles/written-by-christine/the-spoon-theory/
3. "All Might," *My Hero Academia*, S1, Ep12. Adult Swim, June 19, 2016. Television.
4. "Unrest - Facts about ME / Chronic Fatigue Syndrome." *Unrest*, October 4, 2017, https://www.unrest.film/s/Unrest-UK-factsheet-final-04-10-17.docx
5. *Unrest*. Dir. Jennifer Brea. September 22, 2017. Documentary.
6. "One for All," *My Hero Academia*, S3, Ep11. Adult Swim, June 16, 2018. Television.

5. FRIENDSHIP AND FIRE EMBLEM

1. *Fire Emblem: Path of Radiance*. GameCube, Nintendo, 2005. Video game.

2. Skarratt, Leanne. "Friendships and Chronic Illness." *Soul Over Sickness*, October 22, 2018, https://souloversickness.com/relationships/friendships-and-chronic-illness/

6. A DEPRESSED WOLF

1. *Final Fantasy VII: Advent Children.* Dir. Tetsuya Nomura. Square Enix, 2005. Film.
2. Palmieri, Emily. "Advent Children: What's Beneath the Fan Service." *Extra Life*, May 26, 2017, https://community.extra-life.org/articles.html/extra-life-news/communitycontent/advent-children-what%E2%80%99s-beneath-the-fan-service-part-1-r991/
3. Ackerman, Courtney. "Learned Helplessness: Seligman's Theory of Depression (+ Cure)." *Positive Psychology*, March 24, 2018, https://positivepsychology.com/learned-helplessness-seligman-theory-depression-cure/
4. "Chronic Illness and Depression." *Cleveland Clinic*, January 17, 2017, https://my.clevelandclinic.org/health/articles/9288-chronic-illness-and-depression

7. IN SICKNESS AND UNHEALTH

1. Rowling, J. K. *Harry Potter and the Prisoner of Azkaban*. London: Bloomsbury, 1999.
2. Since I wrote this chapter, J.K. Rowling has revealed herself to be anti-trans. This is sadly ironic, since I'm referencing her books to talk about confronting stigmas. I've been sitting in tension with the nostalgia and love I have for the Harry Potter books and disagreeing with the author's harmful views. I left this chapter as it is because I still think Lupin's story speaks volumes about the destruction that othering someone can do. It's telling that the character Rowling created—one who represents a kind, caring, and wise mentor to Harry—would not stand for the stigmas the author herself perpetuates.
3. Rowling, J. K. "Remus Lupin." *Wizarding World*, August 10, 2015, https://www.wizardingworld.com/writing-by-jk-rowling/remus-lupin
4. Rowling, "Remus Lupin."
5. Hirsch, Michele Lent. *Invisible: How Young Women with Serious Health Issues Navigate Work, Relationships, and the Pressure to Seem Just Fine.* Boston: Beacon Press, 2018.

6. Lynne, Kira. *Aches, Pains, and Love: A Guide to Dating and Relationships for Those with Chronic Pain and Illness*. Canada: Moppet Press, 2016.
7. Lynne, Kira. *Aches, Pains, and Love.*
8. Rowling, J. K. *Harry Potter and the Half-Blood Prince*. London: Bloomsbury, 2005.
9. Rowling, J. K. *Harry Potter and the Half-Blood Prince.*

8. THE QUESTION OF CHILDREN

1. "Asylum of the Daleks." *Doctor Who*, S7, Ep1. BBC, September 1, 2012. Television.
2. "Asylum of the Daleks." *Doctor Who.*
3. Mustard, Jenny. "Why I Don't Want Kids." YouTube, August 6, 2016, https://www.youtube.com/watch?v=bHM1giWU8ag
4. Gil, Britney. "No, You Don't Always Love Kids Once They're Yours." *Refinery29*, April 8, 2019, https://www.refinery29.com/en-gb/not-having-kids-parents-abandonment

9. WOMEN. SEX. THE MOON.

1. "Aunt Irma Visits." *The IT Crowd*, S1, Ep6. Channel 4, March 3, 2006. Television.
2. Segert, Liz. "Women more often misdiagnosed because of gaps in trust and knowledge." *Association of Health Care Journalists*, November 16, 2018, https://healthjournalism.org/blog/2018/11/women-more-often-misdiagnosed-because-of-gaps-in-trust-and-knowledge/
3. Chen, E. H. et al. "Gender disparity in analgesic treatment of emergency department patients with acute abdominal pain." *PubMed*, May, 2008, https://www.ncbi.nlm.nih.gov/pubmed/18439195
4. Dusenbery, Maya. *Doing Harm: The Truth About How Bad Medicine and Lazy Science Leave Women Dismissed, Misdiagnosed, and Sick*. New York: HarperOne, 2018.
5. Norman, Abby. *Ask Me About My Uterus: A Quest to Make Doctors Believe in Women's Pain*. New York: Bold Type Books, 2018.
6. Norman, Abby. *Ask Me About My Uterus.*
7. Glantz, M. J. et al. "Gender disparity in the rate of partner abandonment in patients with serious medical illness." *PubMed*, November 15, 2009, https://www.ncbi.nlm.nih.gov/pubmed/19645027

8. Loofbourow, Lili. "The female price of male pleasure." *The Week*, January 25, 2018, https://theweek.com/articles/749978/female-price-male-pleasure

9. Sorensen, James et al. "Evaluation and Treatment of Female Pain: A Clinical Review." *Cureus*, March, 2018, https://www.ncbi.nlm.nih.gov/pmc/articles/PMC5969816/

10. As of 2021, I have been tentatively diagnosed with endometriosis (a specialist diagnosed me based on symptoms, and we're trying other treatments before we resort to surgery). So huzzah that I have a name for the issue and a diagnosis. Boo that the first three or four doctors I told about my pain ignored me and never tested for it. And boo that it's incurable. Endometriosis is the worst, friends. It's right up there with all the other chronic illnesses. They're all the worst. That is all.

11. "Aunt Irma Visits." *The IT Crowd.*

12. Lichtman, Judith et al. "Sex Differences in the Presentation and Perception of Symptoms Among Young Patients with Myocardial Infarction." *Circulation*, February 20, 2018, https://www.ahajournals.org/doi/full/10.1161/circulationaha.117.031650

10. FUEL FOR ANXIETY

1. "Horizons." *Dirk Gently's Holistic Detective Agency*, S1, Ep1. BBC, October 22, 2016. Television.

2. "Horizons." *Dirk Gently's Holistic Detective Agency.*

3. Rowling, J. K. *Harry Potter and the Deathly Hallows.* London: Bloomsbury, 2007.

4. Meeks, Rachel. "When Chronic Pain Leads to Post-Traumatic Stress Disorder." *The Mighty*, August 12, 2016, https://themighty.com/2016/08/how-chronic-illness-can-lead-to-post-traumatic-stress-disorder/

11. IF ONLY I HAD MORE FAITH

1. Roth, Veronica. *Carve the Mark.* New York: HarperCollins, 2017.

2. This chapter has changed slightly from its original version in the first edition of *Super Sick*. I wanted it to be more accessible to people who aren't religious while still remaining true to my personal beliefs. Of course, I can't stop you if you want to skip it completely! However, I hope that all readers will find some nuggets of encouragement here.

3. Bowler, Kate. *Everything Happens For a Reason: And Other Lies I've Loved*. New York: Random House, 2018.
4. Roth, Veronica. *Carve the Mark*.
5. Yancey, Philip. *Where Is God When It Hurts?* Grand Rapids: Zondervan, 1990.
6. Roth, Veronica. *Carve the Mark*.
7. Keller, Timothy. *The Reason for God*. New York: Penguin Books, 2018 (originally published 2008).
8. "Nightcrawler." *X-Men*, S3, Ep18. Fox, May 13, 1995. Television.
9. Virant, Katie Willard. "Cultivating Gratitude while Living with Chronic Illness." *Psychology Today*, November 12, 2018, https://www.psychologytoday.com/us/blog/chronically-me/201811/cultivating-gratitude-while-living-chronic-illness

12. THE MASS EFFECT OF RELIGION

1. *Mass Effect 2*. Windows PC version, BioWare, 2010. Video game.
2. Weeks, Patrick. "Kepral's Syndrome and Cystic Fibrosis: A Request from a BioWare Writer." *FextraLife* forum post, June 19, 2011, https://fextralife.com/forums/t492760/keprals-syndrome-and-cystic-fibrosis-a-request-from-a-bioware-writer/
3. Whitman, Sarah M. "Pain and Suffering as Viewed by the Hindu Religion." *The Journal of Pain*, Vol. 8, No. 8, August, 2007, http://www.uphs.upenn.edu/pastoral/events/Hindu_painsuffering.pdf
4. Whitman, Sarah M. "Pain and Suffering."
5. Melina, Remy. "Spirituality Helps Chronically Ill Men and Women Differently." *LiveScience*, October 29, 2011, https://www.livescience.com/16788-spiritual-support-benefits-chronic-illness.html
6. Carter, Sherrie Bourg. "Helper's High: The Benefits (and Risks) of Altruism." *Psychology Today*. September 4, 2014, https://www.psychologytoday.com/ca/blog/high-octane-women/201409/helpers-high-the-benefits-and-risks-altruism
7. *Mass Effect 3*. Windows PC version, BioWare, 2012. Video game.

13. TO HAVE IT OVER WITH

1. Deaver, Jeffery. *The Bone Collector*. New York: Penguin Random House, 1997.
2. Deaver, Jeffery. *The Bone Collector*.

3. Pederson, Cathy L. et al. "Assessing depression in those who are chronically ill." *Counseling Today*, March 7, 2018, https://ct.counseling.org/2018/03/assessing-depression-chronically-ill/

14. SUPERHEROES ARE SICK

1. Tolkien, J. R. R. *The Fellowship of the Ring*. London: HarperCollins, 2014 (originally published 1954).
2. McCracken, L. M. "Learning to live with the pain: acceptance of pain predicts adjustment in persons with chronic pain." *PubMed*, January, 1998, https://www.ncbi.nlm.nih.gov/pubmed/9514556
3. Tait, Stephanie. *The View from Rock Bottom*. Eugene, Oregon: Harvest House Publishers, 2019.

ACKNOWLEDGEMENTS

My thanks go out to everyone who contributed a piece of themselves to this book, including but not limited to the following people:

All my fabulous alpha and beta readers: Kyle, Casey, Joy Beth, Julia, Christine, Steve, and Lindsay. For your copious notes and encouragement, I am forever in your debt.

My trio of editors—Erin Straza, Kyla Neufeld, and Alex Mellen—you rock!

Matt, for coming up with the super title! See what I did there, Matt?

Fay Onyx, for writing a stellar foreword for a fellow disabled nerd you barely knew!

My parents, for never leaving me alone in a hospital and for advocating on my behalf.

Lisa and Mark, for never making me feel ashamed of being sick. Kyle and Marilyn—ditto.

People of the Hearth and Incantatem, for making me

feel welcome and accepted, and understanding when I don't show up.

All the friends and family who have supported me and made me feel loved.

My husband, Jordan, who never lets me feel ashamed about my illness and offers never-ending encouragement. Also, for leaving me alone to write this book even when he wanted to play video games with me.

Every person I interviewed who gave their time and vulnerability to share their experiences: Elisabeth, Niko, Hannah, John, Doug, Emily, Mitch, Nina, Derek, Kate, Lindsay, Amy, Joy Beth, Sara, Sara Jane, Jason, Elizabeth, Allison, Aaron, Jen, Sarah, Holly, and Sharon. You are all superheroes.

And to all the people suffering from chronic pain and illness—you are not alone.

SICK FICTIONAL HEROES

If you are looking for examples of characters with chronic pain or illness in pop culture, here is a non-exhaustive list. Some I mention in the book, others I do not.

The lines tend to blur between chronic illness, chronic pain, and disability, but I focus on illness and pain or discomfort. My list weighs heavily toward science fiction and fantasy because, well, it's me. I keep an updated version of this list on my website, aealexander.com.

- **Allen Francis Doyle**, *Angel* (TV) — chronic headaches.
- **All Might**, *My Hero Academia* (anime) — respiratory damage.
- **Amanda Brotzman**, *Dirk Gently's Holistic Detective Agency* (TV) — Pararibulitis.
- **Andy Bernard**, *The Office* (TV) — Irritable Bowel Syndrome.
- **Anemone**, *Eureka Seven* (anime) — headaches and nosebleeds.

- **Athena Cykes**, *Ace Attorney: Dual Destinies* (video game) — ultrasensitive hearing and sensory overload.
- **Ava Starr, a.k.a. Ghost**, *Ant-Man and the Wasp* (movie) — chronic pain.
- **Aza Ray**, *Magonia* by Maria Dahvana Headley (novel) — lung disease.
- **Beatrix**, *Battleborn* (video game) — terminal disease.
- **Callum Hunt**, *The Iron Trial* by Cassandra Clare and Holly Black (novel) — injured leg.
- **Carswell Thorne**, *Cress* by Marissa Meyer (novel) —blindness.
- **Cloud Strife**, *Final Fantasy VII* (video game) — Mako poisoning and Geostigma.
- **Collem West**, *The Blade Itself* by Joe Abercrombie (novel) — chronic headaches.
- **Cyra Noavek**, *Carve the Mark* by Veronica Roth (novel) — chronic pain.
- **Eliwood**, *Fire Emblem: Blazing Sword & Sword of Seals* (video games) — debilitating illness.
- **Frodo Baggins**, *The Lord of the Rings* by J. R. R. Tolkien (novels/films) — chronic pain from a knife wound.
- **Greer Sonnel**, *Bloodline* by Claudia Gray (Star Wars novel) — Bloodburn syndrome.
- **Gregory House**, *House* (TV) — chronic pain from muscle death.
- **Harper**, *A Curse So Dark and Lonely* by Brigid Kemmerer (novel) — cerebral palsy.
- **Inara Serra**, *Firefly* (TV) — unnamed illness.

- **Izumi Curtis**, *Fullmetal Alchemist & Fullmetal Alchemist: Brotherhood* (anime/manga) — chronic illness from missing organs.
- **Jane Foster, a.k.a. Thor**, *The Mighty Thor* (comics) — cancer.
- **Jeremy Jamm**, *Parks and Recreation* (TV) — Irritable Bowel Syndrome.
- **Jushiro Ukitake**, *Bleach* (anime) — an illness like tuberculosis.
- **Kaori Miyazono**, *Your Lie in April* (anime) — ALS.
- **Konno Yuuki**, *Sword Art Online* (anime) — AIDS.
- **Laura Roslin**, *Battlestar Galactica* (TV) — cancer.
- **Laphicet**, *Tales of Berseria* (video game) — the Twelve Year Sickness.
- **Lincoln Rhyme**, *The Bone Collector* by Jeffery Deaver (novel) — quadriplegia.
- **Linh Cinder**, *Cinder* by Marissa Meyer (novel) — cyborg.
- **Maria Robotnik**, *Sonic Adventure 2* (video game) — Neuro-Immuno Deficiency Syndrome.
- **Morinth**, *Mass Effect 2* (video game) — a genetic disorder where she kills anyone she mates with.
- **Ninten**, *Earthbound Beginnings* (video game) — asthma.
- **Nux**, *Mad Max: Fury Road* (movie) — tumours and fevers.
- **Puck**, *Alpha Flight* (comics) — constant pain.
- **Raistlin Majere**, Dragonlance series by

Margaret Weis and Tracy Hickman (novels) — unnamed illness.

- **Raoden**, *Elantris* by Brandon Sanderson (novel) — cursed so that injuries never heal.
- **Raven Reyes**, *The 100* (TV) — chronic pain from nerve damage.
- **Remus Lupin**, Harry Potter series by J. K. Rowling (novels/films) — lycanthropy.
- **Rena Hirose**, *Ace Combat 3: Electrosphere* (video game) — Silverstone disease.
- **Rhys**, *Fire Emblem: Path of Radiance* (video game) — unnamed chronic illness.
- **Rin**, *Fruits Basket* (anime) — stomach ulcers.
- **Sand dan Glokta**, *The Blade Itself* by Joe Abercrombie (novel) — chronic pain.
- **Satine**, *Moulin Rouge* (movie) — tuberculosis.
- **Sayo Mutou**, *Rurouni Kenshin* (anime) — tuberculosis.
- **Shannon Rutherford**, *Lost* (TV) — asthma.
- **Simon Phillips**, *Fringe* (TV) — chronic headaches and nausea.
- **Stephen Strange**, *Doctor Strange* (film) — damaged hands.
- **Tali'Zorah**, *Mass Effect 2* and *3* (video games) — weak immune system and dextro-amino acid chirality.
- **Taimi**, *Guild Wars 2* (video game) — disease similar to multiple sclerosis.
- **Thane Krios**, *Mass Effect 2* and *3* (video games) — Kepral's Syndrome.
- **Tony Stark, a.k.a. Iron Man** (movies/comics) — heart condition.

- **Wade Wilson, a.k.a. Deadpool**, *Deadpool* (movies/comics) — cancer and chronic pain.
- **Yonah**, *NieR* (video game) — the Black Scrawl.

When you're frequently sick, you tend to watch a lot of TV. At least, I do. Here's a non-exhaustive list of feel-good shows that I recommend for when you're too tired to do anything else.

- *Avatar: The Last Airbender.* Nickelodeon, 2005–2008. Animated fantasy.
- *Brooklyn Nine-Nine.* Fox/NBC, 2013–present. Comedy.
- *Buffy the Vampire Slayer.* The WB/UPN, 1997–2003. Supernatural drama.
- *Castle.* ABC, 2009–2016. Crime drama.
- *Chuck.* NBC, 2007–2012. Action/spy comedy.
- *Community.* NBC / Yahoo! Screen, 2009–2015. Sitcom.
- *Dirk Gently's Holistic Detective Agency.* BBC America/Netflix, 2016–2017. Supernatural dramedy.

- *The Dragon Prince.* Netflix, 2018–present. Animated fantasy.
- *Doctor Who.* BBC, 2005–present. Sci-fi.
- *Eureka.* Syfy, 2006–2012. Supernatural comedy.
- *Farscape.* Sci-Fi Channel, 1999–2003. Sci-fi.
- *Final Space.* TBS/Adult Swim, 2018–present. Animated sci-fi.
- *Firefly.* Fox, 2002. Sci-fi.
- *The Flash.* The CW, 2014–present. Superhero.
- *Futurama.* Fox/Comedy Central, 1999–2013. Animated sci-fi.
- *Galavant.* ABC, 2015–2016. Fantasy musical.
- *Gilmore Girls.* The WB/The CW, 2000–2007. Comedy drama.
- *The Good Place.* NBC, 2016–present. Supernatural comedy.
- *The Guild.* YouTube, 2007–2013. Comedy.
- *Hunter x Hunter.* Nippon Television, 2011–2014. Fantasy anime.
- *The IT Crowd.* Channel 4, 2006–2013. Comedy.
- *iZombie.* The CW, 2015–2019. Crime drama.
- *Jane the Virgin.* The CW, 2014–2019. Romantic dramedy.
- *The Legend of Korra*. Nickelodeon, 2012–2014. Animated fantasy.
- *Life in Pieces.* CBS, 2015–2019. Sitcom.
- *Lost in Space.* Netflix, 2018–present. Sci-fi.
- *Merlin.* BBC One, 2008–2012. Fantasy.
- *Modern Family.* ABC, 2009–present. Sitcom.
- *My Hero Academia.* Adult Swim, 2016–present. Superhero anime.

- *Mystery Science Theater 3000.* Comedy Central et al. 1988–present. Sci-fi.
- *The Office.* NBC, 2005–2013. Sitcom.
- *Once Upon a Time.* ABC, 2011–2018. Fantasy.
- *The Orville.* Fox, 2017–present. Sci-fi.
- *Parks and Recreation.* NBC, 2009–2015. Sitcom.
- *Psych.* USA Network, 2006–2014. Comedy/mystery.
- *RWBY.* Rooster Teeth, 2013–present. Animated fantasy.
- *Samurai Jack.* Cartoon Network/Adult Swim, 2001–2004, 2017. Animated fantasy.
- *She-Ra and the Princesses of Power.* Netflix, 2018–present. Animated fantasy.
- *Speechless.* ABC, 2016–2019. Sitcom.
- *Stargate SG-1.* Showtime/Sci Fi, 1997–2007. Sci-fi.
- *Stargate Atlantis.* Sci Fi Channel, 2004–2009. Sci-fi.
- *Star Trek: Discovery.* CBS, 2017–present. Sci-fi.
- *Star Trek: The Next Generation.* First-run syndication, 1987–1994. Sci-fi.
- *Star Wars: The Clone Wars.* Cartoon Network/Netflix/Disney+, 2008–present. Animated sci-fi.
- *Star Wars Rebels.* Disney XD, 2014–2018. Animated sci-fi.
- *Supergirl.* CBS/The CW, 2015–present. Superhero.
- *Sword Art Online.* Adult Swim, 2012–2014. Sci-fi anime.

- *Timeless.* NBC, 2016–2018. Sci-fi.
- *Veronica Mars.* UPN/The CW/Hulu, 2004–2019. Mystery drama.
- *Video Game High School.* FreddieW, 2012–2014. Comedy.
- *Warehouse 13.* Syfy, 2009–2014. Supernatural comedy.
- *White Collar.* USA Network, 2009–2014. Crime drama.

RELAXING VIDEO GAMES

Here are some games that I consider calming, whether because of the gameplay, beautiful art style, lovely music, or thoughtful themes. I've played many of these when I want to relax or when I'm tired but my body just won't let me fall asleep.

- *Abzû.* Microsoft Windows, PlayStation 4, Xbox One, Nintendo Switch. Giant Squid Studios, 2016. Adventure.
- *Age of Empires II.* Microsoft Windows, Mac OS, PlayStation 2. Ensemble Studios, 1999. Real-time strategy.
- *Animal Crossing.* Nintendo 64 et al. Nintendo, 2001. Social simulation.
- *Astroneer.* Microsoft Windows, Xbox One, PlayStation 4. System Era Softworks, 2019. Adventure.
- *Brothers: A Tale of Two Sons.* Xbox 360, Microsoft Windows, PlayStation 3, PlayStation

4, Nintendo Switch. Starbreeze Studios, 2013.
Adventure.

- *Child of Light.* Microsoft Windows, PlayStation
  3, PlayStation 4, Wii U, Xbox 360, Xbox One,
  Nintendo Switch. Ubisoft, 2014. Role-playing
  platformer.
- *Chrono Trigger.* Super NES, PlayStation,
  Nintendo DS, Microsoft Windows.
  Square/Square Enix, 1995. Role-playing game.
- *Dragon Age: Inquisition.* Microsoft Windows,
  PlayStation 3, PlayStation 4, Xbox 360, Xbox
  One. BioWare, 2014.
- *Fe.* Microsoft Windows, Nintendo Switch,
  PlayStation 4, Xbox One. Zoink, 2018. Action-
  adventure.
- *Final Fantasy IX*. PlayStation, Microsoft
  Windows, PlayStation 4, Nintendo Switch,
  Xbox One. Square, 2000. Role-playing game.
- *Final Fantasy XIII.* PlayStation 3, Xbox 360,
  Microsoft Windows. Square Enix, 2009. Role-
  playing game.
- *Flower.* PlayStation 3, PlayStation 4, Microsoft
  Windows. Thatgamecompany, 2009.
  Adventure/art.
- *GRIS.* macOS, Microsoft Windows, Nintendo
  Switch, PlayStation 4. Nomada Studio, 2018.
  Platform-adventure.
- *Hollow Knight.* Microsoft Windows, macOS,
  Linux, Nintendo Switch, PlayStation 4, Xbox
  One. Team Cherry, 2017. Action-adventure.
- *Journey.* PlayStation 3, PlayStation 4, Microsoft
  Windows. Thatgamecompany, 2012. Adventure.

- *Kerbal Space Program.* Microsoft Windows, macOS, Linux, PlayStation 4, Xbox One. Squad, 2015. Space flight simulation.
- *Limbo.* Xbox 360, PlayStation 3, Microsoft Windows, Linux, Xbox One, PlayStation 4, Nintendo Switch. Playdead, 2010. Puzzle-platformer.
- *Minecraft.* Microsoft Windows, macOS, Linux. Mojang, 2011. Sandbox/survival.
- *Myst.* Microsoft Windows, Mac OS, PlayStation, PlayStation Portable, Nintendo DS/3DS. Cyan, 1993. Adventure/puzzle.
- *Okami.* PlayStation 2, Wii, PlayStation 3, Microsoft Windows, PlayStation 4, Xbox One, Nintendo Switch. Clover Studio, 2006. Action-adventure.
- *Ori and the Blind Forest.* Microsoft Windows, Xbox One, Nintendo Switch. Moon Studios, 2015. Platform-adventure.
- *No Man's Sky.* PlayStation 4, Microsoft Windows, Xbox One. Hello Games, 2016. Action-adventure/survival.
- *RiME.* Microsoft Windows, Nintendo Switch, PlayStation 4, Xbox One. Tequila Works, 2017. Puzzle/adventure.
- *Slime Rancher.* Microsoft Windows, macOS, Linux, Xbox One, PlayStation 4. Monomi Park, 2017. Life simulation.
- *Stardew Valley.* Microsoft Windows, macOS, Linux, PlayStation 4, Xbox One, Nintendo Switch. ConcernedApe, 2016. Farming simulation/role-playing.

- *Terraria.* Microsoft Windows. Re-Logic, 2011. Action-adventure/sandbox.
- *The Legend of Zelda: Breath of the Wild.* Nintendo Switch, Wii U. Nintendo, 2017. Action-adventure.
- *The Legend of Zelda: Ocarina of Time.* Nintendo 64, GameCube. Nintendo, 1998. Action-adventure.
- *The Legend of Zelda: The Wind Waker.* GameCube. Nintendo, 2002. Action-adventure.
- *Shadow of the Colossus.* PlayStation 2. SCE Japan Studio, 2005. Action-adventure/puzzle.
- *Thomas Was Alone.* Microsoft Windows, PlayStation 3, Linux, Mac OS, Xbox One, PlayStation 4, Wii U. Mike Bithell, 2012. Puzzle-platformer.
- *Undertale.* Microsoft Windows, Mac OS, Linux, PlayStation 4, Nintendo Switch. Toby Fox, 2015.
- *Warcraft III.* Microsoft Windows, Mac OS. Blizzard Entertainment, 2002. Real-time strategy.
- *The Witness.* Microsoft Windows, PlayStation 4, Xbox One, macOS. Thekla, Inc., 2016. Puzzle.

BONUS MATERIAL: FIVE MORE SICK HEROES AND THEIR FRUSTRATIONS

When this book was first released in 2020, I visited several blogs to write about some of my favourite sick heroes who didn't get mentioned in the main text of this book. Some of those short blog posts are compiled below, in which I spotlight Laura Roslin from *Battlestar Galactica*, Raven Reyes from *The 100*, Raoden from *Elantris* by Brandon Sanderson, Wade Wilson from *Deadpool*, and Jane Foster from *The Mighty Thor* comics.

———

Often, when a book or movie represents a disability or illness, the entire thing is *about* that illness; think *Forrest Gump* or *The Fault in Our Stars*. These characters' identities are entirely swallowed up by their disabilities. In other shows, characters with illnesses are only there on the sidelines to "inspire" the protagonist, in the way that Tiny Tim's only purpose in *A Christmas Carol* is to be pitied by Scrooge.

Writers have also excluded characters with disabilities from stories due to the idea that once you're disabled or chronically ill, you're done. You're no longer a hero until you have found a cure or have "overcome" your disability.

As someone with a chronic illness, I appreciate it when I see three-dimensional protagonists who have conditions and are learning to deal with them while taking part in a larger narrative—characters like the following five fictional heroes who have particularly inspired me due to their methods of coping.

1. LAURA ROSLIN AND PERSEVERING

Laura Roslin is abruptly promoted from Secretary of Education to the President of the Twelve Colonies at the beginning of *Battlestar Galactica*. Throughout the show, she faces incredibly difficult decisions with calm and poise as murderous robots, the cylons, threaten to destroy the fleet of human survivors. On top of battling for the lives of humanity and the stress of survival, Laura has terminal breast cancer. She has to deal with exhaustion, pain, treatments, side effects, and knowing that she's fighting for a future that she will not live long enough to see.

Perhaps, you're thinking, "What a great role model! She must inspire and encourage everyone in the fleet!"

Haha. Well. If you've watched *Battlestar Galactica*, then you know that no one in the show is a great role model (except maybe Helo, but I digress). Every character is flawed, makes mistakes, and makes terrible decisions. Laura is no exception. Not everyone loves her. In fact, quite a few people hate her. She's *human*. And that's how characters with disabilities and illnesses should be portrayed: as human. (Of course, alien or cylon is fine, too.)

As the show goes on, Laura's condition deteriorates but her determination does not. In her position, I would be tempted to give up the presidency and find a corner to curl up and be sick in, but Laura spends her time fighting for the other souls in the fleet. Laura's cancer does not swallow up her identity. It doesn't take over the story. It doesn't define her. And this is why I love her character so much.

2. RAVEN REYES AND PRESSING ON

Raven Reyes from CW's *The 100* is the spunkiest, cleverest, and most creative character among the group of teenagers attempting to survive on post-apocalyptic Earth. She doesn't let anything stop her. Rules, she'll break 'em; mechanical problems, she'll solve 'em; her boyfriend's death, she'll grieve and carry on. Until she's shot in the spine, that is. After surgery, Raven has to live with chronic pain due to nerve damage, and it almost destroys her.

Anyone who lives with chronic pain knows the toll it takes on your mind and body. It's exhausting. It's frustrating. And when there's no end in sight, it's difficult to find hope or purpose in life.

In Season Three, Raven responds to her pain by refusing to slow down or admit she can't do all the things she used to. She feels like accepting her condition would be admitting she is weak, and resists that—until she's presented with a chip she can swallow that will take away her pain. At first, she responds with scorn at this "miracle cure," but then she gives in because she just wants the pain to stop. And who can blame her?

Many shows would end her character arc here, with a cure, and let her go on with a "normal," healthy life where she can run around stabbing enemies in the face like the rest of the show's characters. Except, *The 100* doesn't do that. The chip works, sort of. It removes Raven's pain, but at the cost of her memories and agency. In the end, she accepts that her disability is a part of her, that she has purpose and hope even with her limitations. Her technological brilliance allows her to defeat the season's villain, disability and all.

I love her arc, because those of us with disabilities and chronic pain don't get miracle cures, either. If we think people like us can't contribute to the exciting adventures in a science fiction or fantasy novel, we're wrong. Raven proves that.

3. RAODEN AND FINDING HOPE

In Brandon Sanderon's first published novel, *Elantris*, Raoden is cast into the city of Elantris after being taken by the Shaod, a transformation that used to change his people into gods but now turns them into something more akin to zombies.

"Every pain… every cut, every nick, every bruise, and every ache—they will stay with you until you go mad from the suffering," an Elantrian named Galladon informs him upon his arrival.

Elantrians can't die, but they also can't heal. Even the

pain of a stubbed toe stays with them forever. As simple cuts and scrapes add up (never mind if they accidentally break a bone), their pain increases, and eventually they go crazy from it.

Sanderson's descriptions of constant pain and the depression the Elantrians suffer strike home for me. It's incredibly difficult to describe how chronic pain impacts your brain unless you've experienced it yourself. It's a monster that drains your life away.

"What purpose do we have besides suffering?" Galladon asks.

"We need to convince ourselves we can go on... If we can restore even a tiny bit of hope to these people then their lives will improve drastically," Raoden says.

Hope is something that those of us with chronic pain desperately search for—not necessarily hope for a cure, but hope that life means something and that we can find peace despite our suffering. This is what Raeden brings to the Elantrians; he creates a community of people who support each other and uses distraction as a coping mechanism. He gives the people tasks to do, like rebuilding the city's crumbling structures. He buries himself in books, which helps keep his mind off the pain. This is a familiar tactic to me, as I often read books, watch TV, and play video games to keep my mind off of my own pain.

Raoden's perseverance in searching for hope reminds me to do the same. I don't always find it, especially when I've spiralled into depression, but I remember what that hope felt like and I can rest and try searching for it again tomorrow.

4. WADE WILSON AND CONFRONTING SHAME

Sure, maybe you shake your head at Wade Wilson in *Deadpool* for leaving his girlfriend, Vanessa, because he doesn't want her to watch him die. It doesn't make sense! She *wants* to be there for him, cancer diagnosis and all. It's not his choice to make!

Maybe you are even more annoyed when he is cured (cured of the cancer, that is, not of the chronic pain), but still doesn't return to her because he's disfigured and ashamed. He sees himself as a monster and doesn't think he deserves to be with her, even though she loves him.

I was annoyed with his decision, too. It's easy to be mad at someone else instead of confronting this exact same tendency in myself.

I, too, am ashamed of my illness. I feel like I'm worth less than others, because they can do things that I can't. *They* don't need to take a three hour nap in the afternoon because they're too exhausted to go back to work. *They* don't need to rush to the bathroom with pain squeezing their gut at the drop of a hat. *They* don't need to cancel on their friends for the umpteenth time because they're too sick to leave the house.

Why would anyone choose me, when they could have a relationship with someone healthy?

It's taken a long time to accept that my illness is part of me, but it doesn't define me. It has nothing to do with my value as a person. People have chosen to love me, sickness and all, and it's not my job to "protect" them from me or reject them because I think they could do better.

I am valuable, I am loved, just the way I am, and so are you. Take it from Deadpool and don't make the same mistakes he did. Or else the whole world will taste like Mama June after hot yoga.

5. JANE FOSTER AND VALUING YOURSELF

In The Mighty Thor comics (and the upcoming *Thor* movie), Jane Foster takes Mjölnir and becomes Thor. What's awesome about this is that she has the powers of a god—the superest of super heroes—and she has a chronic illness.

Superheroes are usually the epitome of strength and health, characters who I have trouble empathizing with. *I can never be like that,* I think as I watch Wonder Woman running around saving people. She doesn't falter in exhaustion just from leaving the house to get groceries, after all.

But Jane Foster *is* like that. She has cancer. And she still does amazing things in both her god and mortal form.

> "I am Jane Foster," she narrates in The Mighty Thor #1. "And believe it or not, I'm also The Mighty Thor. Though right now I'm not feeling particularly mighty. Right now I'm just trying not to die."

In her Thor form, Jane doesn't have cancer; she is only plagued by the illness when she reverts back to her human body. So why doesn't she stay in the Thor form all the time, you ask? If I was her, I don't know if I could give up feeling healthy for the weakness, the puking, the exhaustion, the Chemo brain. But she does because "not even the Mighty Thor is a match for every challenge. If I'm going to save everyone I know and love from the specter of war… then Jane Foster has a job to do as well."

That's right, Jane Foster, the sick and unhealthy version, has value. Worth. Purpose. Her story doesn't just end because she's sick. Her Thor form isn't an answer or cure for her sickness—in fact, it's more of a problem for it, because becoming Thor clears out the chemo from her body, but doesn't cure the cancer.

So often, I feel like I'm worthless unless I'm cured, but Jane Foster's story tells me that's a lie. My value isn't tied to being healthy. I matter and I have a voice just the way I am, and so do you.

BONUS MATERIAL: AN INTERVIEW WITH ALLISON ALEXANDER

This interview was conducted by Kriti Khare of *Armed with a Book*, and first appeared on her blog during my book tour. Thanks, Kriti!

KK: How important have representations of disability been in your life, especially when you were a kid?

AA: As a kid, I didn't consciously notice characters with disabilities or compare myself to them. Most of the characters I would have seen were Tiny Tim types—there to be pitied or to inspire another character. I didn't think of myself like that. The first time I compared myself to a character on TV was when I saw the anime *Fullmetal Alchemist* as a teenager. In the show, Izumi Curtis is a feisty alchemist who has an illness that makes her cough up blood. I was enthralled because she was sick *and* she was a badass hero taking an active role in the story. I loved seeing a character who wasn't on the sidelines, whose identity wasn't swallowed up by her illness.

KK: I remember her! I enjoyed her role in the series. And talking about *Fullmetal Alchemist*, that series has so many outstanding characters. That makes me want to rewatch it now. Are there any other memorable characters from the series for you that you connected with on a personal level?

AA: I normally like side characters more than protagonists, but I love Edward Elric. He's stubborn and determined to get his brother's body back. He also has this strong moral code he refuses to break. He's gone through so much suffering, including losing a literal arm and leg, but uses the bad experiences to do good. Riza Hawkeye also reminds me of myself because she's so quiet, calm, and loyal—sometimes to a fault! She's so disciplined that she rarely relaxes. I've been practicing going easier on myself so I've gotten a little better at it, but that's still a struggle for me.

KK: What are some misconceptions or misrepresentations you have found about chronic illness and disability in fiction?

AA: I came up with a checklist for when I am analyzing fiction and for writers to use when they are creating disabled characters. It includes the whole "we're only there to be pitied or inspire others" thing. Another misconception is that disability is a "problem" that needs to be cured. You can download the checklist and read about a positive example (one of my favourite characters —Toph Beifong from *Avatar: The Last Airbender*) by signing up for my newsletter on aealexander.com!

KK: That is super handy, thank you Allison! What led you to create such a list?

AA: I'm an acquiring editor at a small press that publishes sci-fi and fantasy, so I'm constantly looking for positive representation in the book submissions we receive. I realized a checklist might be useful for writers to look over, so I compiled a list of the things I look for when I encounter disabled characters.

KK: What are some ways in which readers and reviewers can help bring more awareness about characters with disabilities in fiction?

AA: Be aware when you read a positive example of disability in fiction and that this is to be celebrated. Follow disabled writers and review books that feature these characters. Educate yourself on what a positive example is and why it's so valuable to those of us with disabilities and chronic conditions.

KK: Can you give us an example of a positive representation?

AA: I just read *A Curse So Dark and Lonely* by Brigid Kemmerer and I appreciated its inclusion of a disabled protagonist. Harper has cerebral palsy and is not defined by her disability. The book's plot does not revolve around her condition. She's not there to inspire another character. She's a feisty young woman who gets drawn into another world and plays a significant role in the fate of a fantasy kingdom. There are characters who think that she's useless and needs to be protected because of her condition, but she refuses to be put in that box.

A lot of representation in fiction isn't perfect, and Kemmerer's book is no exception. One of the critiques is that Harper could be switched out for an able person and the story would have been very similar. I would have liked to see her cerebral palsy cause her a few more problems in the narrative and to manifest itself as more than just a limp. But this book is a step in the right direction, proof that heroes don't have to be physically perfect or healthy.

KK: I have yet to read *A Curse So Dark and Lonely*, and I am so glad you mentioned it. Bumping it on my list! The one character that comes to my mind is Ella from *The Illuminae Files* by Amie Kaufman. Ella is not a protagonist but plays such an important role in the book with her hacker skills and intelligent thinking. She is paralyzed from the waist down and wears an oxygen mask; in spite of that, she fights alien parasites and humans. The book is written in the form of logs and transcripts of surveillance footage and still does a good job of showing Ella's strengths.

Your book's blog tour actually reminded me that not all chronic illnesses are obvious to identify. You shared about Raven from *The 100* on my blog and it was eye opening to me that I had totally missed the fact that her constant pain is chronic pain now. Similar to trigger warning and content notes, sometimes experience is what helps us notice certain things in fiction and media. What are your thoughts about this?

AA: I wouldn't have clicked so much with Raven's desire to swallow the chip and be rid of the constant pain if I hadn't experienced chronic pain myself. Chronic illness is difficult to understand if you haven't experienced it yourself, and you can definitely overlook it in fiction and reality. A lot of people with chronic conditions also aren't comfortable talking about it—we never know who will believe us or what other people's responses will be, and it's not our duty to "educate" people. I've had people tell me, after reading my book, how shocked they were when they realized the amount of pain and stress I go through.

I also may not have realized just how underrepresented disabilities are in fiction if I hadn't started researching it for my book. I wanted a positive example for each chapter that related to a particular topic (e.g. anxiety, depression, worthlessness, etc.) and realized just how few my options were. That led me to start noticing and appreciating positive examples wherever I found them. It was an unconscious appreciation before (for example, I loved the character Laura Roslin from *Battlestar Galactica* but didn't really connect the dots about why her character resonated with me so much until later). I didn't think much about disabled characters in fiction when I was younger because *I never saw them*. They weren't an option. Now that I know they are, I love being able to put myself in the shoes of a chronically ill superhero and I want more opportunities to do so!

KK: Just looking has opened a whole new world. Many books have been made into movies and I am wondering if you have noticed whether chronic illness

representations translate well from the book to screen since they are very different mediums. Your analysis of *Final Fantasy* characters in *Super Sick* was really helpful to me and, though I have not played the game, it showed how interactive media can present these themes too.

AA: I think any medium can include characters with chronic illnesses. I suspect it is often a challenge, especially for invisible illnesses. It's easier to feature a healthy, fit hero. Books do have the advantage of getting into the character's head; that's where a lot of my battles with chronic illness take place. Other media has to show that struggle in different ways.

Video games are a huge part of my life and they include another level of putting myself in a character's shoes. Some of the games that have impacted me most haven't featured chronic illness specifically, but include a character working through grief and loss: *RiME*, *GRIS*, and *Final Fantasy IX* were particularly visceral experiences for me in this way. There is something cathartic about progressing through gorgeously drawn levels and seeing the character you control experience grief. In story-based games, I really appreciate when a playable character has an illness. In *Super Sick*, I mention Cloud from *Final Fantasy VII* and Rhys from *Fire Emblem: Path of Radiance*. There are a few others I'm aware of—*Ace Attorney*'s Athena Cykes has sensitive hearing, *Earthbound Beginnings*' Ninten has asthma, and *Sonic Adventure 2*'s Maria Robotnik has Neuro-Immuno Deficiency Syndrome—and I hope to encounter more.

KK: This has been an amazing conversation, Allison! Thank you so much for taking time out for answering my questions and sharing your experiences.

ABOUT THE AUTHOR

Allison Alexander writes articles, edits sci-fi and fantasy
books, and plays video games
the rest of the time. She is the
incurable author of *Super Sick:
Making Peace with Chronic
Illness*, an honest (and occasionally sarcastic) testimony
about living with a chronic
illness. Allison makes her home
in Hoth, a.k.a. Winnipeg,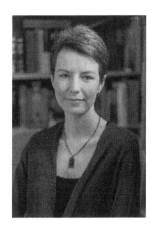
Manitoba, with her husband and their giant collection of
tabletop RPG manuals. You can also find her chasing
bokoblins in Hyrule, traipsing with elves in Middle-earth,
or blogging at aealexander.com.

goodreads.com/authoraealexander
twitter.com/allisonexander
instagram.com/allisonexander

Manufactured by Amazon.ca
Bolton, ON